THE JOURNEY'S END

THE JOURNEY'S END

An Investigation of Death and Dying in Modern America

MICHAEL DORING CONNELLY

ROWMAN & LITTLEFIELD
Lanham • Boulder • New York • London

Published by Rowman & Littlefield
An imprint of The Rowman & Littlefield Publishing Group, Inc.
4501 Forbes Boulevard, Suite 200, Lanham, Maryland 20706
www.rowman.com

86-90 Paul Street, London EC2A 4NE

British Library Cataloguing in Publication Information Available

Library of Congress Cataloging-in-Publication Data

Names: Connelly, Michael, 1953- author.
Title: The journey's end : an investigation of death and dying in modern
    America / Michael Doring Connelly.
Description: Lanham : Rowman & Littlefield, [2023] | Includes
    bibliographical references and index.
Identifiers: LCCN 2022039829 (print) | LCCN 2022039830 (ebook) |
        ISBN 9781538175484 (cloth) | ISBN 9781538175491 (ebook)
Subjects: LCSH: Death--Social aspects. | Terminal care. | Hospice care.
Classification: LCC HQ1073 .C658 2023 (print) | LCC HQ1073 (ebook) |
        DDC 306.9--dc23/eng/20220830
LC record available at https://lccn.loc.gov/2022039829
LC ebook record available at https://lccn.loc.gov/2022039830

CONTENTS

FOREWORD

When Michael Connelly asked me to write the foreword to this book, I privately thought, "Wow, does the world need another book on death and dying?" However, since I have known Michael for nearly thirty years and am one of his biggest fans, I thought, "Well let me do a deep dive here and see what happens." I am so glad that I followed my instincts.

In the United States, we believe that death is an option—and have foolishly poured untold resources, time, and energy into futile attempts at preventing death. Sadly, this has resulted in a terrible set of circumstances.

Fortunately, *The Journey's End* is the best single treatise on understanding this conundrum I have ever read. It offers a roadmap for our society to provide better and more humane care at the end of life. I am not surprised that Michael Connelly, a prominent national leader and past chair of numerous national and international boards in healthcare, was able to cut through the complexity and controversy surrounding this crucial topic.

I have always found the language of death objectionable. Our culture praises as heroes those who choose to fight death to their last breath while consuming expensive, futile treatments. What nonsense! Does this mean that others who accept their fate of dying without resorting to expensive care are not equally as brave? Michael confronts this contradiction.

This book expertly weaves heartfelt advice with serious scholarship. It references nearly every major book on death and dying and even incorporates primary sources such as the famous stoic philosopher Seneca. I was particularly enamored by the four phases of elderhood, going from awareness to the consequences of our health choices, to intentionality, to action. This reminds me of the young Elizabeth Kübler-Ross decades ago laying out the four stages of coming to grips with death. Importantly, *The Journey's End* brings a much-needed, fresh perspective to this ancient problem.

Much like this book, I've long argued that fee-for-service medicine is the root of all evil in the health system. It needs to go, and this author has a sound plan for its demise.

Clinically it is my experience that many of my colleagues feel obligated to do everything to forestall death, often resulting in the unintentional torture of the patient and the involved family. I have seen this so many times at the bedside in both the critical care unit and in the general patient wards of Jefferson Health, a place that has been my academic home for more than three decades.

Michael's timing for this book is excellent. Our great country has suffered a million deaths from COVID-19, the largest per capita death rate of any developed nation in the world. The COVID-19 pandemic shined a brighter light on all of these challenges and demonstrated that no one is immune to the death trap. Indeed, many of these early deaths were in communities of color and among people with limited resources and dwindling economic means.

We are facing skyrocketing inflation and the potential for a bankrupt Medicare trust fund as early as 2026. At the same time, we are figuratively teetering on the precipice as our system of delivering healthcare services begins to collapse under its own weight. In my view, COVID-19 should accelerate our embrace of the prescriptions for healthcare reform in *The Journey's End*.

As a medical educator, I've always felt that deep reform would entail two things: first, a modified approach to medical education; and second, a broader approach to creating the doctor of the future—a physician who can accept death at the appropriate time and serve as a guide to families. Sadly my own personal experience mirrors my clinical-life experience. Dealing with the death of my parents was a traumatic experience not because of their demise but because of the rabbit hole of useless medical care that they fell into. It took my physician wife and me, with all of our resources, to literally grab her parents out of a similar rabbit hole in order for them to have a good death.

Frank Davidoff and Paul Batalden were right when they noted that doctors, nurses, pharmacists, and others in healthcare all have two jobs every day.[1] Job 1 is the clinical job they were trained to do. And job 2 is working hard to always find a way to improve job 1. Sadly most clinicians have no training in job 2, and therefore the system is a self-perpetuating machinery that now consumes 20 percent of our GDP with nearly $4 trillion in annual spending. Most experts agree that about a third of all that spending is of no value.[2]

Fittingly this book brings these opportunities for improvement to life with vivid illustrations of wasteful and counterproductive care. I believe that everyone would benefit from reading *The Journey's End* and especially its conclusion, which makes pragmatic—and readily implementable—suggestions for reform. I also hope this book will change the conversation about death by making it more humane, honest, and just.

David B. Nash, MD, MBA
Founding Dean Emeritus
The Dr. Raymond C. and Doris N. Grandon Professor of Health Policy
The Jefferson College of Population Health
Spring 2022

ACKNOWLEDGMENTS

Completing this book would never have been possible without the critical comments and expert advice of my son Quinn Michael Connelly. Quinn was instrumental in translating my ideas into more coherent prose while constantly looking for valuable research and quotes to support my arguments. Quinn's overall influence on my thinking (or my lack of thinking) and the book's completion was profound.

Second, I want to recognize Jonathan Agronsky, my editor, who helped me tremendously to organize my random thoughts into a logical sequence of chapters. The way he sequenced my ideas into topics and chapters was brilliant. He also helped me create a more compelling voice by pushing me to include personal stories in each chapter.

Dr. David Nash has been one of my clinical mentors for decades. Dr. Nash's long-term dedication to improving the quality of patient care is inspirational. His advocacy for improving the quality of care helped inspire and encouraged me to write this book. His kind words in the foreword are deeply appreciated. Next is Dr. David Leach, a national authority on physician education, who gave me encouragement and support for my ideas in this book from the beginning of the journey. He also provided several powerful stories for the text. Father Myles Sheahan, MD, as an ethicist and geriatrician was also an essential supporter and text reviewer. Chris Lowney, a former Jesuit, retired JP Morgan executive, and bestselling author, kindly reviewed the manuscript. His critical advice and perspective were invaluable.

Finally three more physicians helped me throughout the book. Dr. Richard Afable, a practicing clinician and healthcare executive, offered valuable insights into the book. Dr. Robert Clemency, a close friend, was kind enough to review the manuscript at various phases and provide valuable feedback. And Dr. David Babbitt was my resource for understanding the difficulties physicians face when guiding a patient through difficult care choices. He also provided relevant patient stories.

My financial expert was David Nowiski, a seasoned financial expert with significant knowledge in physician compensation. His expertise was critical in helping me wade through the complexity of this subject matter. Sr. Doris Gottemoeller, RSM, provided an insightful review of the manuscript with excellent suggestions. My close friend for the past thirty years Sr. Marie Hartmann, RSM, has mentored me throughout my career. She is an inspiration to my faith and has been my lifetime counselor.

Let me close by thanking my beloved wife of forty-seven years for her support and creative thinking on a book topic that is not exactly popular. This book would not have been possible without the loving support of my entire family: Chris Connelly, Meredith Connelly Koch, Quinn Connelly, and my three fabulous grandchildren Graham Koch, Grace Koch, and Malcolm Connelly. Hopefully their future will be enhanced by implementation of the recommendations in this book.

INTRODUCTION

[We need to] radically reimagine a better system for death and dying.[3]

The more sophisticated our society becomes, the more we resist death. Every person's end-of-life journey is different, yet our medical care models are rigid and controlling. What we need are models of care that adapt to each individual's changing needs, models that offer alternatives in terms of settings and services.

But what is needed even more than a change in care models is a shift in attitude. Specifically, we should stop trying to medicalize death because it is, and should be, a natural process. That said, determining the right care for each patient while also preserving their autonomy and dignity is a challenge. It becomes even more difficult when the patient is frail, confused, or has otherwise lost agency.

This is why knowing a patient's preferences is so crucial. Few if any caregivers really know the care their patient truly desires. Why? Because we don't candidly discuss end-of-life care. This inability to address death is a shame because facing mortality is one of life's most important skills—especially in old age. Even so, most of us spend our life avoiding even the thought of our final days.

As this book will argue, grappling with the reality of death has both practical and philosophical benefits. Indeed, it gives us closure, freedom, and a sense of purpose. Or in the words of Michel de Montaigne, one of the Renaissance's most prominent philosophers, "Premeditation of death is premeditation of freedom. . . . He who has learned how to die has un-learned how to be a slave. Knowing how to die frees us from all subjection and constraint." (*The Laws of Human Nature*, Robert Greene, 586).

The *Lancet*, a renowned medical journal, has published a ground-breaking project on death and dying. The research, which was conducted by a worldwide commission of experts, suggests that we need to recover our appreciation for the value of death in society.[4] Perhaps more fundamentally we need to release ourselves from the social expectation that in old age we are obligated to fight against death with all that medicine has to offer.

As this book will show, a societal appreciation for death is long overdue. In fact, an unfortunate shift in attitudes toward death has occurred over the last several decades. Today dying is no longer a familial experience but rather a cold, clinical, and medical ordeal. The *Lancet* study argues the balance between death and dying needs to be restored. In other words, the process of dying should be owned by individuals and family members with support from health professionals—instead of the other way around.

Put simply, modern medicine overreaches in its attempts to fend off death. In fact, we have gone so far as to medicalize grief. This excessive focus on clinical intervention at the end of life is costly and comes at the expense of other social needs. The report calls on everyone to develop "death literacy" because people have lost the skills, traditions, and values that our predecessors used to deal with death.

Fortunately, a key focus of *The Journey's End* is developing this death literacy and owning how we wish to face death. It is an in-depth investigation of the experience of death and dying in the United States. This book also provides recommendations on how this investigative knowledge can be used to improve healthcare for the elderly and dramatically reduce healthcare expenses.

The U.S. healthcare system has a narrow view of caring for patients in old age. That view focuses on extending life with technology and not managing or supporting the patient's social needs. As such, it is likely we will spend the last years of our lives in long-term care facilities and our final weeks in a hospital ICU. These environments are not conducive to intimate family gatherings where some of life's most cherished moments are shared. Dying at home, peacefully, surrounded by family is almost impossible in our technocratic world.

Fittingly, the thesis of this book is that in old age it is more important to *understand* your life than *extend* it. While this thesis is seemingly simple, its implications are profound. Moreover it is precisely these implications that deserve our attention.

Understanding the U.S. healthcare system and its incentives is essential in today's world if families wish to find quality care for their elderly. For example, have you ever wondered why your physician hardly has time to talk with you or understand your concerns? Or why the health system doesn't offer you a single physician to help coordinate your multiple health conditions or answer your questions? The dysfunctionality of healthcare is well-trodden territory, but the root causes of the problems surrounding these questions are ripe for investigation. The root causes of these problems deserve our attention. Consider the following:

1. Why have we created a system with economic incentives that prevent physicians from getting to know their patients or communicating with one another about their shared patients? These incentives have given us fragmented healthcare.
2. Why is there an obtuse billing and coding system that drives physicians to focus only on quantifiable treatments? This obsession with measurement over common sense has given us a physician-compensation system that is destroying the patient-physician relationship.
3. Why as a society are we unwilling to embrace the reality of trade-offs in developing health policy? Specifically, why do we choose to pay for futile and costly attempts to avoid death but refuse to pay for social support services that are effective, needed, and much less expensive?

Overall these three root cause issues drive the dysfunction of U.S. healthcare.

While the existing system shortchanges everyone, it is the elderly who bear the brunt of this burden. The elderly suffer most from chronic illnesses and, therefore, are most harmed by fragmented healthcare. That said, the status quo of ineffective and expensive care for the elderly is not the only option. We as a society can take a different approach by changing the system's incentives and embracing natural death. Moreover, we can achieve this change through comfort care instead of fruitless attempts to "cure" old age. This change in direction will require more awareness and death literacy from everyone.

A natural death means that at some point we choose to accept that we are old enough to die. The concept of being old enough to die is not easy to embrace and deserves some unpacking. Death has value and is often misunderstood. In our cynical and overly clinical age, it isn't easy to reflect on the value of death, but that kind of honest introspection is precisely what we need. Accepting one is old enough to die means no longer feeling obligated to pursue diagnostic treatment or burdensome medical care. There are many sound reasons to pursue this course of care at some point in life. However, this is a personal choice not a third-party choice. Unfortunately, it often becomes a third-party choice due to our loss of agency near the end of life.

The Journey's End seeks to help individuals and their families manage their healthcare choices in the final phase of life by better understanding their options. As a wise man once said, "Life is pleasant. Death is peaceful. It's the transition that's troublesome." I hope this book proves a guide for that troubling transition.

1

PREPARING FOR THE
LAST PHASE OF LIFE

Death—it's our greatest fear. But this fear has effects we
are not even aware of. . . . We live in a culture that takes
denial to the extreme, banishing the presence of death
as much as is possible. If you go back hundreds of years,
you could not have failed to see people die in front of
you. . . . Death had a presence. It was constantly there.
And so people were thinking about it all the time. And
they had religion to help soothe the idea of their mortality.
Death had a presence. . . . We now live in a world where
it's the complete opposite. We have to repress the very
thought of it. . . . Nobody ever talks about it.

—Robert Greene, *The Daily Laws*

No one knows when, exactly, they will die. Yet we expend tremendous amounts of energy avoiding death. Why? The answer is
simple: because we fear it.

Dying is not merely a medical issue. Dying is about understanding
your life and who you are as a person. Unfortunately in today's clinical age,
these qualitative concerns are often diminished if not entirely dismissed.
My belief is that in order to avoid unnecessary suffering and spending
at the end of life, each of us needs to take more responsibility for how
we face death. In our waning years, we face many challenges such as
deciding how to use the healthcare system. Deciding how we use the healthcare system in old age is a crucial part of facing death. For many people,
taking more personal responsibility for healthcare decisions may translate
into worthwhile rewards.

1

Ironically, medical specialization and technological advances have made the process of dying *more* not *less* troublesome.

Dying today faces broad, systemic challenges. While our modern healthcare system focuses narrowly on curing illness, as we age our chronic diseases become increasingly incurable. In such circumstances, healthcare providers too often respond by treating our symptoms because there is no cure for old age. Our inability to face this reality often results in endless and expensive treatments that do more to extend misery than prolong meaningful life. Compounding this problem is the complex interplay between patients, families, guardians, and healthcare professionals. As we age, incompetence becomes more commonplace. Incompetent patients are unable to make decisions about their care. Consequently, difficult care choices burden families and health professionals alike. In far too many cases, these decision makers take the safe route of doing everything possible. Unfortunately, this safe route ignores the immense personal, physical, familial, and financial trade-offs associated with doing everything clinically possible.

Many healthcare professionals realize doing everything possible is wasteful and harmful, but the healthcare system ties their hands. They fear being sued for not taking heroic measures to prolong a patient's life; they may even fear criminal prosecution. Or perhaps it is their professional training that has taught them to be overly reliant on curing options. Economic incentives are another force driving patients toward overtreatment. All in all, our culture prioritizes a clinical treatment approach over a compassionate family caring approach.

The consequences of this overly clinical culture are as predictable as they are problematic: healthcare spending has escalated at an average rate of 2 percent *above* inflation for more than *three decades*.[5] The compounding effect of this rate of inflation hurts everyone. A significant portion of this spending is on futile end-of-life (EOL) care. It should come as no surprise, then, that healthcare spending accounts for almost 20 percent of our economy—almost double that of any other industrialized democracy. Until we find a way to fix our broken healthcare system, including changing our approach to EOL care, this figure will continue to rise. These steadily rising healthcare costs consume our economy and diminish our country's ability to invest in other social needs like education, children, infrastructure, and the most marginalized in society.

No one disputes that these matters are complex and personal. Our reluctance to discuss death and dying, however, is not an excuse for inaction. Every American deserves to die with dignity and without risking bankruptcy or burdening future generations. So how do we begin to take action and make progress in addressing these issues? The first step is trying to better understand—and face—our fear of death.

In his book *The Unbroken Thread*, Sohrab Ahmari discusses our society's loss of tradition. As part of that discussion, he explores how to face death with wisdom. He acknowledges that death is "life's ultimate barrier" and that it shouldn't be surprising that our modern outlook on life is utterly opposed to death.[6]

Ahmari convincingly argues that attempting to defeat death is a mistake. In other words, our cultural attitude of wanting to live forever is unwise. Life is a journey, and all journeys must have an end. Ahmari turns to Stoicism for advice and shows how Stoic philosophy can offer wisdom in the face of death. Specifically, he offers four lessons from Seneca, the famous Roman Stoic philosopher.

The first lesson is that we are less likely to fight death if we intentionally prepare ourselves for it. "Those who desperately cling to life often do so at an exorbitant cost to their dignity."[7] Our natural reaction to facing death is to panic—seeking to do everything possible to stay alive. In old age, this attitude can be a serious mistake because an artificially extended life can be worse than death.

Seneca's second lesson is that fearing death is really pointless. Death is everywhere, and the potential causes of death—hurricanes, pandemics, violent crime, a fall, a car accident—can occur at any time. It makes no sense to fear the inevitable, especially in old age. As Seneca explains, "To live life fearlessly, then, we need to make peace with the fact that death is ever present."[8]

The third lesson is that death is an equalizer—it happens to everyone. Seneca argues that seeking to live forever is arrogance. "[Dying] establishes a democracy of sorts among people of all generations," Seneca wrote. "It happened to your father, your mother, your ancestors, everyone before you, everyone after you. An unbreakable sequence, which no effort can alter."[9] Of course accepting death is difficult, but not accepting—or outright denying—death implies a certain sense of superiority.

The fourth and final lesson is that death gives meaning to life. An excessively long life can become a curse—especially when it is dependent on intrusive medical care. Seneca thought of it this way: "No journey is without an end point. . . . Just as with storytelling, so with life: it's important how well it is done, not how long."[10]

In sum, Seneca offers us these four lessons to help us overcome our natural fear of death and to motivate us to prepare for our own death.

Another important step in this preparation is to envision our own approach to the last phase of life. After a lifetime of pushing ourselves to be efficient and productive, how do we re-orient ourselves during this extended time in life? One way to embrace our new freedom in old age is by reflecting on, and contemplating, topics we never had time for when we were busy working. While there will be things we can no longer do as we age, old age does offer us the opportunity to find a new path forward.

Many try to fight and resist their decline given the alluring technology available through modern medicine. But it's worth asking, Is this a worthy fight? That is a choice each of us must make individually, and there is no universally applicable, right answer. Yet learning more about these options has its benefits. For instance, learning about what modern medicine can (and cannot) offer you is important.

Moreover we do not fully appreciate the importance of preparing ourselves for this responsibility. While the day we are born and the day we die are perhaps the two most important events in our life—these two events offer us a useful study in contrast. When it comes to the birth of a child, we go through extensive preparation. We change our living habits, we buy new furniture, and make all kinds of safety adjustments to our home. We also educate ourselves on how to prepare for the birth process and for parenthood.

By contrast, what do we do to prepare for our own death? For far too many people, the answer is nothing. My argument is that we need to prepare for death as seriously as we prepare for a newborn. Unfortunately, most of us will not adequately prepare. We live longer—in some cases decades longer. These added decades will involve significant interaction with the healthcare system. Those interactions will come at vulnerable moments and will call on our families to make challenging choices—life-and-death choices. Those choices will impact how we live in those decades and how we die. It is also likely that we will lose our mental capacity to make our own choices. Interestingly, one of the most pressing problems in the financial world today is elderly clients squandering their savings through incompetence and ignorance.

Our lack of preparation for death raises the question What if we are squandering our final years by refusing to accept the realities of mortality?

It wasn't long ago that most people died of natural causes, at home, with their family. In my opinion, these deaths were far better for everyone involved. They were substantially less expensive too. As this book will explain, this holistic approach to dying is difficult to achieve in today's high-tech healthcare system.

First, we must acknowledge the fact that at some point in life we are old enough to die. There is no formula or specific age for this realization—it requires wisdom and reflection. It is probably one of life's most personal choices and will most likely be an incremental one. As we start becoming frail in old age, we can choose to accept that it no longer makes sense to try and cure what can't be cured. After this realization we can shift the focus of our healthcare away from prevention, intervention, and sophisticated treatments. Instead we can move toward a model of care that focuses on support and comfort. We might view healthcare treatment as a resource we want to conserve and avoid because it is no longer that beneficial. Death is inevitable, and at some point there are no more cures.

This is a difficult personal choice, and people are free to pursue all that modern medicine has to offer. That said, an artificially prolonged life involves trade-offs and costs that deserve thoughtful consideration. This book is about helping you become better informed. It is also intended to motivate you to become a more responsible decision maker— and not falling victim to the U.S. healthcare system's default settings.

Embracing the end of life can be rewarding. This period of life will include physical diminishment along with personal growth and development. Your diminishment will include physical losses in hearing, sight, flexibility, endurance, memory, and strength. Your personal growth and development will come from the opportunity to use your life's accumulated knowledge, skills, and wisdom to reflect on the meaning of your life and to share your wisdom with others.

That said, this stage of life presents us with trade-offs. Will we learn to embrace everything aging has to offer us, the good and the bad? Or will we spend those extra years resisting it?

My advice is to be *intentional* about how you make use of your extended life—which is a gift. Your life will most likely be longer, and have more health complications, than you anticipate. As we age, our body's ability to recover from setbacks will diminish.

The healthcare system's approach to caring for the elderly is to evaluate each illness separately. (Note: This approach is, in part, driven by the coding system for billing.) As such, we have separate drugs, treatments, and often physicians for each illness. For the frail elderly, this approach to care can be particularly confusing. This phenomenon has come to be described as *fragmented care*.

It may seem obvious, but it bears repeating: in old age, we are in decline. Our immune system weakens, we lose mental capacity and muscle strength, and we become increasingly vulnerable to chronic conditions like arthritis, rheumatism, high blood pressure, clogged arteries, and incontinence. The root cause of these conditions, of course, is old age. Attempting to treat illnesses, individually and one by one, without acknowledging the overall problem—which is the physical decline of old age—is a major oversight of our healthcare system.

In clinical terms, this transition is referred to as losing our *homeostasis*. A less-technical way to think about this concept is to understand that as we age our ability to recover from injury declines. A simple fall can be fatal.

It's important to keep in mind that medical care for a frail, elderly person can cause injury unintentionally. These treatments, tests, and procedures negatively affect the elderly more than they impact healthy adults.

The more frail and vulnerable we are, the more injurious these procedures may become. This is an important point to remember when you are offered medical treatment and diagnostic procedures in old age. The way medical research works is that medical treatments are tested on younger and more vibrant individuals. Therefore the physician's confidence in using a test or procedure is skewed by results from a younger population.

Let me illustrate this point with a patient story. A good friend, whom I will call Mary, was ninety-two years old and in relatively good health.[11] She discovered blood in her stool and was understandably concerned. She was able to quickly get an appointment with a gastroenterologist to advise her on how to proceed. He advised her that the bleeding was most likely from the pain medications that she was taking for her severe arthritis. Nonetheless, the physician recommended a more elaborate diagnostic test to rule out cancer. (For better or worse, physicians are trained to be safe rather than sorry, and this can result in ordering too many tests.)

As part of this precautionary principle, Mary had an esophago-gastroduodenoscopy scheduled. This procedure requires an unpleasant preparation process similar to the one for colonoscopies. For younger individuals, this may be a routine, albeit unpleasant, experience but one that is acceptable because of its documented benefits in catching cancer early. For Mary, this procedure was more challenging. Her arthritis was so severe that the pain in her spine prevented her from lying flat. She actually was sleeping in a recliner, not a bed, because of that pain. When Mary arrived at the hospital for the procedure, they tried to transport her lying flat on a cart. That was not going to happen since it would have been extremely painful. Eventually they found a work-around solution.

For Mary, given her frail condition and advanced age, the benefits of this routine procedure were less clear. In other words, the procedure took a significant toll on her body. It was an unpleasant experience, and she was nauseous and foggy for a week afterward. The benefits were also questionable. Her pain medication was the most likely cause of her bleeding, and she could have avoided the procedure by changing her pain medications instead. Nevertheless she agreed to this procedure because she wanted reassurance that she was cancer free. However, even if she did have cancer, it is unlikely much could be done for her given her frailty at age ninety-two. Fortunately the original diagnosis was correct, and she did not have cancer.

In an effort to be safe rather than sorry, her doctor had recommended this procedure. But was this procedure worth it? While she had initially thought so, after experiencing the drawbacks of the procedure firsthand, Mary concluded it was not worthwhile. Of course, this episode illustrates the high cost of safety especially for the frail and elderly population.

To be clear, this outcome was not the physician's fault. As professionals, physicians are generally under appreciated. They have dedicated their lives to medicine and take great personal risk in caring for patients.

That said, patients need to take more responsibility for deciding what treatments and diagnostic tests make sense for them.

The critical question, then, is why have we designed a healthcare system that makes it so difficult for caregivers to discuss these issues with their patients thoroughly? This is a complicated question and one that is explored throughout this book.

However, this chapter is about how we choose to embrace the end of life. It is also about using these final years to deepen our understanding of life. This journey begins by addressing our biological and psychological fear of dying. Dying is part of life, yet our fear of death drives behavior that may not be beneficial to us or our family. One person recently told me it was fortunate they were retired because otherwise they wouldn't have enough time to go to all of their doctor appointments. That raises the question Do you want to spend your last decade going to doctor appointments? Or do you want to spend that time with family and friends? Trade-offs like these are a recurring theme throughout this book.

Ideally, elderly patients should be treated like unique individuals and not as a laundry list of illnesses, symptoms, and medications. Recognizing that elderly individuals are different from one another, and taking into account their life story, habits, and relationships, will greatly improve their care. Also, supporting public policies that allow patients to stay in their home would in most cases be a better choice. This option would put patients first by bringing support services to them rather than making them go to an institution. Moreover, denying the elderly the opportunity to share their wisdom by isolating them in institutions is poor public policy. Overall, it will require both individual and societal change to make this EOL approach to care a reality.

This book attempts to guide the reader through the four phases of elderhood: (1) awareness, (2) learning the consequences of our healthcare choices, (3) intentionality, and (4) action.

The first phase is awareness of what we need to know about healthcare. Modern medicine focuses heavily on technology and complex treatments. Given this, it is critical that we be aware of the importance of comfort care as an alternative option. While the realities of healthcare in old age may be grim, it is very beneficial to be aware of what to expect.

The second phase is learning the likely consequences of our healthcare choices. My premise is that healthcare is focused on remedies for specific problems instead of on care for the whole person—for instance, specific problems like reduced cardiac function, cancer, or kidney failure. Treatments for these conditions, in most cases, don't focus on your overall health or stage in life. In old age, these treatments are in many cases not worth the trial and tribulation. Moreover, these treatment choices have consequences beyond the individual. For example, what are the impact of these treatments on healthcare spending? On our own pain and suffering? On our family and on future generations? This second phase examines the consequences of healthcare choices in old age.

The third phase is intentionality. Once you better understand what to expect from healthcare in old age, you need to decide how you want to use it. It is important to understand there is a high probability that you may lose or have diminished mental capacities before you die. As such, it's critical to make your intentions known, in writing, well in advance. Informed consent is an essential aspect of determining your intentions. The key here is to make an informed decision about your healthcare choices before it is too late.

The fourth phase is action—namely, what actions can individuals, institutions, and society as a whole take to advance this new vision for end of life. Chapters 1–11 of this book focus on what the individual needs to know about healthcare and how they might better prepare themselves. Chapters 12–19 focus on the public policies needed to facilitate a new vision of EOL care for the elderly.

As a society we can avoid the default option of ineffective and expensive care with a natural death. Moreover, we can achieve this through comfort care instead of trying to cure ourselves of old age. Dying a natural death means accepting that at some point, we are old enough to die. This is a very difficult decision, and each person should be free to make or not make that decision for themselves. The implications of such a decision are that we may no longer seek any active medical treatment other than pain management. The ability to effectively make this decision is enhanced through preparation and education. One way to help with this decision is to reframe our choices at the end of life with wisdom in mind rather than science alone as our guiding light.

The goal of this book is to help individuals and families find a better path on this journey. This book differs from others on EOL care in three ways. First, it integrates economics with the clinical decision-making process. Economics is a trade-off we cannot disregard. Second, it examines issues from multiple disciplinary angles including cultural, clinical, legal, political, economic, and ethical perspectives. This approach helps identify the root causes of the problems we face in healthcare. This root-cause analysis is then converted into practical suggestions for improving EOL care. Third, this book argues the design of U.S. healthcare delivery is destroying the fundamental physician-patient relationship. Fixing this core relationship is the key to fixing healthcare. Therefore, concrete recommendations are offered to change the system in various ways to improve physician-patient communication and better inform patients about their best healthcare choices.

I have been in the trenches of healthcare for over forty years, running hospitals and large health systems. It has been a rewarding and educational journey, and it has exposed me to virtually every aspect of healthcare. Over my career I've grappled with hundreds of difficult patient cases, countless complex regulations, and difficult decisions involving painful trade-offs. Personally I've also lived through my own healthcare scare and journeyed through EOL care with family and close friends. My learning from these experiences, both personally and professionally, is that EOL care reform is the key to improving the healthcare system in this country. Addressing the issue of fragmented healthcare with practical solutions is at the heart of this opportunity.

The audience for this book is any family dealing with healthcare issues for the elderly and health policy leaders. It includes anyone—especially older adults—interested in learning how to improve their interactions with the healthcare system. The book begins by focusing on the individual: What experiences should we expect from elderhood? How does the healthcare system think and function in relation to the elderly? The book then transitions to wider healthcare reform and how to improve EOL care. Throughout the book you will learn how the health system works. This knowledge will facilitate your understanding of what is happening and why it is happening. Healthcare is complicated but I will walk you through it one step at a time.

2

AGONY AS THE DEFAULT OPTION

If you do not change direction, you may end up where you are heading.

—Chinese philosopher Lao Tzu[1]

Too often when the American healthcare system is confronted with a gravely ill elderly patient, its default response is to use high-tech medical devices such as ventilators, dialysis machines, and defibrillators to extend the patient's life. As countless American families already know, the results of this technology-driven approach to EOL care can be devastating. Nowadays, it is all too easy for a dying patient to fall into what I call the "death trap." By this I mean undergoing invasive, discomforting, but ultimately futile medical interventions at the end of life.

Unless explicitly directed otherwise, the healthcare system will ensnare you with excessive and invasive EOL care. I refer to this experience as a death trap because such overbearing care can trap you in a painful dying process.

These measures are frequently taken without patients and families fully comprehending their implications. Rather, as noted by journalist and hospice volunteer Ann Neumann in her 2016 book *The Good Death: An Exploration of Dying in America*, "We often don't so much make decisions as drift into passive indecision and acquiescence to authority, whether that be doctors, nurses or hospital policy."[2]

Although many medical practitioners find this approach to EOL care deeply flawed, no one (so far) has been able to fix it. What frustrates would-be reformers most is this fundamental paradox: Nearly everyone who allows this dysfunctional EOL treatment model continues to believe they are doing the right thing.

U.S. doctors, for example, are educated, trained, and, upon graduation from medical school, required to swear a Hippocratic Oath to preserve life—not end it. When a patient dies while under their care, they may feel that they have failed in their fundamental duty to keep that person alive. On an intellectual level, this seems irrational. People get sick, they get old, they get injured, and they die. Doctors are not necessarily culpable for this inevitable outcome. But doctors are human, and we all know from bitter experience that few accept the feeling of failure.

Medical practitioners, of course, do not operate in a vacuum. In Western society, every human life is deemed precious and thus, by definition, worth saving. It is mainly in America, however, that extending a dying patient's life through medical care is widely considered a virtuous act. Except in those very rare cases in which the patient fully recovers from a deadly illness, prolonging a patient's life in this manner is, in my opinion, anything but virtuous. Let me give you an example of how badly things can turn out when well-meaning clinicians treat a dying patient in a way they believe to be dutiful and correct.

DAVID'S STORY

David retired in his mid-sixties after a successful career as an engineer and inventor. He was a World War II veteran with a distinguished service record. He and his wife, Ellen, lived happily together in the house they had built outside a midwestern city. They loved their home, in which they had raised their daughter. They hoped to spend their golden years there together. For nearly a decade, they lived their dream. Then Ellen died. David, of course, was very sad. But his daughter, Nancy, and his son-in-law, Ed, to whom David was unusually close, visited him often, easing his loneliness. When David was age eighty, however, a problem came up that love alone could not cure: David developed Alzheimer's.

With support from Nancy, Ed, and the home healthcare workers they hired, David was, amazingly, able to remain in his home for another decade. By age ninety, however, he needed around-the-clock supervision and care. Reluctantly, Nancy placed her father in a nursing home for Alzheimer's patients. Fortunately David had been successful in life, so Nancy was able to use his assets to pay the $100,000 plus in annual nursing-home fees. She found additional comfort in knowing that when her father's time came, he would be able to die naturally. David had executed an advance directive (also called a living will), a legally binding medical document in which he stipulated that he did not wish to receive any extraordinary medical interventions at the end of his life. He also had given Nancy medical power of attorney, enabling her to make medical decisions for him if he lost the ability to make them for himself.

After spending nearly two years in the nursing home, David contracted pneumonia. Within days, he was approaching death. The nursing home physician suggested to Nancy that her father be given hospice care, which focuses on making the patient comfortable and pain-free rather than on curing the underlying illness. She agreed. The doctor advised her that without treatment, the pneumonia would probably take her father's life within seventy-two hours. To Nancy, it appeared the doctor was complying with David's advance healthcare directive (AHD), a copy of which she had provided to the nursing home when her father was admitted to the facility.

Following a shift change at the nursing home, a new nurse took over David's care. Upon assessing his condition, she concluded that a round of antibiotics could possibly save him. The attending physician, of course, already knew this. By withholding the medicine, he was giving David a chance to die naturally as was David's stated wish. In retrospect, it appears the nurse either was unaware of David's AHD or chose to ignore it. Without checking with the doctor, which is staff protocol in most medical facilities, she called Nancy directly to obtain her approval for changing her father's treatment. According to Nancy, the nurse did not make it clear to her that the new medicine she proposed giving to her father was an antibiotic that might cure his pneumonia and thus extend his life. It is worth noting that pneumonia can be painful for a patient, and pain medications in these situations are not unusual. Believing the drug treatment would ease David's suffering, she approved it. The nurse then called the doctor, requesting he pre-scribe the antibiotic medicine based on Nancy's approval of the new medication. Mistakenly assuming that Nancy had changed her mind— such last-minute reversals are not uncommon when a loved one is dying—the physician canceled David's hospice care. He ordered the high-powered antibiotics. The drugs knocked out David's pneumonia. However, he still had Alzheimer's and was existing in a world in which he recognized no one, including his family.

I learned about this family's predicament when Ed, who is a close friend of mine, asked me if I thought Nancy should sue the nurse, the doctor, and the nursing home for violating her father's AHD. He said the undesired antibiotic treatment had caused much needless suffering for both David and for them. Ed also suspected that the nursing home might have had an economic incentive to keep David alive. Every year he survived, the nursing home would collect an additional $100,000 from David's dwindling savings to pay for his care and residency. I advised Ed that in the United States it is very difficult to sue a clinician or a medical facility for keeping a patient alive despite the patient's stated wish to die naturally. I also explained that because antibiotics are the medical standard of care for pneumonia, the nursing home doctor and nurse could argue they were *obliged* to give David the potentially life-saving drugs unless instructed to withhold them by David's medical surrogate.

I later reflected on how this unfortunate sequence of events came about and if it could have been avoided. Everyone responsible for David's care played a role in this sad outcome.

The nurse had instigated the crisis by unilaterally initiating the antibiotic treatment and failing to explain clearly to Nancy that the proposed drug treatment could extend her father's life. This is where everything started to go wrong.

Before canceling David's hospice care, the attending physician should have confirmed that the family no longer wanted this patient to die naturally.

As her father's medical surrogate, Nancy should have demanded a clearer explanation of the proposed change in care.

Given the complexity of this disturbing chain of events, Nancy decided not to sue. She did move her father to a different medical facility, but nothing could be done to improve his life. Thus ended a very sad tale with no clear-cut hero or villain and a paradoxical outcome: the unintended sentencing of a frail, elderly, demented patient to two more years in nursing home purgatory by professional healers doing what they mistakenly believed was right.

There are two important takeaways from David's story. First, it shows the importance of having a physician with the time to coordinate and facilitate communication between the doctor and the patient or the patient's surrogate, especially at the end of life. Nothing short of taking time for this level of communication is acceptable when a patient's life—or as in this case, a patient's right to die as he intended—is on the line. Second, it shows the need to make clinicians face some consequences for disregarding a patient's AHD. These situations should be treated as "sentinel events," which would better hold doctors and nurses accountable for ignoring patient directives.

In the healthcare system, the term "sentinel event" refers to making a medical error serious enough to be formally investigated by an independent peer group. An example of a sentinel event in medicine would be wrong-side surgery. In the past, formally citing a clinician for committing an avoidable medical error has proven effective in reducing the incidence of future medical errors. It is also a constructive approach to address this issue that avoids accusations of malpractice. Letting clinicians know they will be held accountable by their peers for ignoring a patient's AHD could fundamentally change their approach to EOL care and save more patients from falling into the death trap.

SAVING THE PATIENT TO DEATH

The lengths to which some doctors will go to keep a dying patient alive would almost seem ridiculous if the results were not so disturbing. To give you an example, John, a professional colleague of mine, told me about the excruciating medical ordeal inflicted on his eighty-eight-year-old maternal aunt Libby less than a week before she died.

"She had spent the past eight years in a nursing home," John told me, "just a dozen miles from the house in the small Western Pennsylvania town in which she had been born and spent most of her life. A series of strokes had confined Aunt Libby to a wheelchair. Her throat muscles were partially paralyzed. She had difficulty swallowing. She could barely speak. But whenever I visited her, she always managed to tell me, 'Johnny, I want to go home.'"

He said his aunt, a retired school nurse, developed sepsis—a systemic poisoning of the bloodstream—when an infection caused by a bedsore on her ankle spread. She was transferred to a local hospital, where an orthopedic surgeon amputated the gangrenous lower portion of the leg in which the infection had begun. He believed he had saved her life. He had consigned her to the death trap.

"I visited her in the hospital following her surgery," John told me:

> She was delirious from the pain-killing drugs they gave her but still clearly in pain. I don't think she recognized me or understood anything I said to her. She died in agony a few days later.
>
> To this day, I don't understand what that surgeon possibly could have been thinking when he cut off her leg. Did he really think Aunt Libby would prefer spending a few more days on Earth in excruciating pain rather than being allowed to pass on naturally?

While this patient story might be an extreme case, it is nonetheless representative of reality. Stories such as these signify the need to put a stop to the unnecessary suffering caused by well-meaning, but tragically misguided, physicians (or families) eager to extend a patient's life regardless of the human or financial cost.

THERE ARE EXCEPTIONS

To be fair, it should be noted that not every medical intervention for a frail, elderly patient turns into a tale of horror. A good friend of mine, Bob, an orthopedic surgeon, told me an amazing story about one of his surgical patients. This story illustrates that age alone does not determine the success of a treatment. The patient's genetics, health status, and state of mind are the key determinants of a successful treatment.

One day Bob received a phone call from a colleague, a cardiologist with an outstanding reputation, asking Bob if he would do a hip replacement on Gwen, a patient of his who was one hundred years old.

> I'll admit, this request took me by surprise. It took me a moment to gather my thoughts because surgery is risky enough even for someone half her age.
>
> "She just needs a new hip," the heart doctor assured me, "so she can continue to enjoy life. She really wants this surgery; I'm sure she'll pull through just fine."

I trusted this doctor's judgment. So I agreed to do it.

Bob successfully replaced Gwen's hip. In the process of meeting her, operating on her, and monitoring her recovery, he got to know her a little better. Everything the cardiologist had said about her, Bob found, was on target. "If anything, she was even more vibrant than I expected," he commented.

Bob said Gwen recovered quickly from the surgery and returned to her surprisingly active lifestyle. Flash forward five years.

"I received a call from Gwen's daughter," said Bob. "She invited me to her mom's 105th birthday party. I happily accepted. At the celebration, Gwen told me, 'Having that hip surgery was one of the best decisions I ever made.' Two years later, I learned she had died of natural causes."

To this remarkable centenarian, going under the knife was merely a bump in the road that barely interrupted her happy journey through the world. She was the proverbial exception to the predictable hazards of old age and a classic example of the indomitability of the human spirit and good genes.

TECHNOLOGY'S UNWITTING ROLE IN THE DEATH TRAP

In 1957, researchers at Johns Hopkins University Medical School led by electrical engineer William B. Kouwenhoven unveiled the first portable external defibrillator, which used electric shocks to restore a steady rhythm to a quivering heart. This precursor to the modern automated external defibrillator (AED) weighed two hundred pounds but it could be wheeled into a stricken patient's hospital room or deployed in an ER.

Dr. Kouwenhoven, a German immigrant to the United States, was also a pioneer in closed-chest cardiac massage, by which oxygenated blood is manually pumped to the brain via chest compressions on a patient whose heart has stopped. Very quickly, this revolutionary new life-saving technique, known as cardiovascular pulmonary resuscitation, or CPR, became the standard of care for any patient experiencing cardiac arrest.

The widespread adoption of the heart defibrillator and CPR, starting more than sixty years ago, fundamentally changed the practice of medicine. It also laid the groundwork for creation of a default EOL care model. The operating principle behind both the AED and CPR was simple: If a life can be saved, save it—even if this means fending off a patient's naturally occurring death for only a few more hours or days.

According to physician and medical researcher Leslie J. Blackhall, MD, CPR, in particular, proved so effective in bringing patients back to life—at least temporarily—it created another problem: deciding when it should be used. In a research paper published in the *New England Journal of Medicine* in November 1987, Dr. Blackhall cited post-intervention survival rates in thirteen studies of more than one thousand CPR–revived patients.[3] "In all these papers," said this researcher, "we see a discrepancy between the initial response rate (16 to 45 percent) and survival until discharge (from the hospital) of 5 to 23 percent."[4]

Her conclusion, after investigating what had brought these patients to the hospital: "It is clear that survival after CPR is related to the underlying illness that leads to the arrest and that patients with certain conditions very rarely survive."[5] Dr. Blackhall noted, for example, that no revived patient with metastatic cancer, acute stroke, sepsis, or pneumonia lived until discharge and that the survival rate for several other serious medical conditions, such as low blood pressure and kidney failure, was only 2 to 3 percent. By contrast, the patients most likely to leave the hospital alive following CPR revival were heart attack victims and patients whose hearts had stopped due to a drug overdose or complications from a medical procedure or anesthesia.[6]

Eventually the poor prognosis for CPR-revived patients suffering from acute illness helped bring about Do Not Resuscitate orders (DNRs), by which patients explicitly or by means of a surrogate elect in advance not to be revived if their heart stops as a part of the natural process of dying.

DNRs became necessary, Dr. Blackhall noted in her research article, because "there is potential harm in CPR in that [revived] patients may be kept alive for days to weeks undergoing painful and dehumanizing procedures with no conceivable medical benefits."[7]

Unfortunately, many medical patients, including those with a terminal illness, do not have a DNR in place—in part because neither they nor their doctors feel comfortable discussing their impending death. As a result, almost everyone who "codes" (stops breathing) in or out of a hospital is almost certain to receive CPR in an attempt to bring them back to life. Knowing this, a good friend of mine, a physician named Richard, intervened in a medical emergency involving his frail, elderly father.

Richard told me he was working at a hospital when he received a frantic call from his mother, informing him that his father couldn't breathe. He immediately surmised that his father, who had cardiac problems, was having a heart attack. He told his mom to call 911. He then beat the ambulance to the house and found his father dead. The paramedics arrived a few minutes later, assessed the patient, and prepared to perform CPR on him. Richard knew that watching the resuscitation effort, which almost certainly would prove futile, would be very distressing for his mother. The worst-case scenario, he knew, would be that his father would be revived and then would spend a few torturous days in an intensive care unit (ICU) before dying again. Not wanting to take the chance that his dad might be caught in the deathtrap, Richard used his authority as a qualified physician to officially declare his father dead. The well-meaning paramedics were forced to step back.

Kenneth A. Fisher, MD, summarizes well in his book *In Defiance of Death* the benefits of rethinking our use of CPR.

> Reducing the use of CPR by 50 percent, eliminating the most futile cases, would increase the long-term survival rate to 20 percent. This single step could save . . . approximately $13 *billion per year*, allow our hospital based physicians to spend more time on patients they can help, and eliminate the suffering of patients who initially survive resuscitation only to spend days to weeks in an ICU before they die.[8]

Here is one more story from a seasoned emergency room (ER) physician in Kentucky that further illustrates the difficulties caused by CPR and our legal system. This physician shared with me his frustration over having to give CPR to patients with documented DNR orders. He indicated hospital lawyers advised him that state law presumed DNRs were invalid in the ER! Families would express to him frustration and question why he was giving CPR to a patient with a documented DNR. He commented he didn't have a logical explanation to give these families. My interpretation of this absurd situation would be that if a patient is seeking care in an ER, they are implicitly withdrawing their DNR. The fact that these patients and their families go to the ER because they are afraid or uncertain what to do is irrelevant. The malpractice-defense world is not comfortable accepting the ambiguity of a DNR as an adequate defense for not reviving a patient in the ER. So doctors in the ER may well be required to ignore a DNR order because they are treating patients seeking emergency care. This may be the logic of the law, but it flies in the face of good common sense.

STICKING AROUND NO MATTER WHAT

Sometimes it is the patient who unwittingly engineers their own EOL debacle. Moreover, it is not unusual for a dying patient, whether fearful of death or not, to insist that his or her doctor keep them alive as long as possible.

"Many people," says physician Jeanne Fitzpatrick, coauthor of *A Better Way of Dying*, "are committed to fighting to the last breath, no matter the circumstances—sentient or not, despite any imaginable level of incapacity, pain or suffering."[9]

While researching her 2010 book along with her sister and coauthor, attorney Eileen Fitzpatrick, Dr. Fitzpatrick says they "talked with people who feel that we are given only one span of life on this planet and that we should not deprive ourselves of a single possible breath. We say, 'More power to them.'"[10]

In *The Lost Art of Dying*, Dr. Dugdale discusses patients' natural resistance to death. Dugdale shares the death experience of Susan Sontag, an activist, bestselling author, and philosophy professor who died in 2004: "Sontag fought death and paid a heavy price. Raging against death, she urged her doctors to continue therapy after she lost most of her lucidity, so great was her fear of her own extinction. Her passion for fighting death was so great that she was never able to say goodbye to her loved ones. She had a lonely death."[11]

Patients' families, particularly adult children, also can help perpetuate the default EOL care model by insisting that the treating physician pull out all the stops to keep their parent alive. This situation often is made even more challenging for the attending doctor by family disagreements. For example, one sibling may advocate for a natural death while another might insist that the doctor use all available means to keep their parent alive. In such cases, the only safe option for the physician, in terms of legal liability, is to do everything—which means, in effect, condemning their patient to the death trap.

The threat of a lawsuit is just one of the many reasons the U.S. healthcare model is stuck in default mode. Another reason is that many terminal patients are simply unaware that they can choose a natural death. They do not know that palliative—or comfort—care and the services of a hospice are available to them. In subsequent chapters, you will learn about some innovative solutions to the problem of patient education on this subject.

RESISTANCE TO CHANGE

Inertia is a powerful force particularly in these life and death situations. Inertia allows the death trap to continue snaring terminally ill patients. The American healthcare system will continue to respond automatically to a dying patient with invasive, life-saving measures unless the patient or the patient's family or surrogate objects. On those rare occasions when our political leaders have tried to alter the default healthcare model, they have been blocked. For a telling example of how politicized the debate over healthcare reform in this country has become, one need only harken back to the cynical attempt by conservative members of Congress to characterize a key aspect of President Obama's 2010 Patient Protection and Affordable Care Act as an attempt to ration healthcare. The opposing lawmakers claimed the president wanted to create bureaucratic death panels to determine an ailing patient's fate. They argued, without providing any supporting evidence, that merely allowing Medicare to reimburse physicians for talking with patients about their EOL care choices, as proposed in President Obama's healthcare reform legislation, was somehow equivalent to the government deciding who will live and who will die. These politicians knew their mischaracterization of the proposal, aimed at scoring political points with voters, would hurt everyone who stood to benefit from this commonsense reform. Yet they persisted with their death panel accusation and won the political showdown.[12]

Six years later, this modest and reasonable proposal eventually became the law of the land. Medicare authorized a new billing code for Advanced Care Planning.[13] For the first time, the government's medical insurance program was officially encouraging primary care doctors to talk with their elderly or chronically ill patients about EOL care options. They did this by allowing physicians to bill for this service. To date, however, only a handful of doctors have taken advantage of this modest reform. As a result, many of the people who could benefit the most from such educational efforts, our country's aging seniors, remain ignorant of their EOL care options and thus vulnerable to the death trap.

Our collective tendency as Americans is to over-consume healthcare services—especially those that are covered by insurance. This tendency has contributed to, and sustained, the death trap. One key lesson of economics is the importance of incentives and constraints. For example, if an expensive, high-tech treatment or procedure costs an insured patient almost nothing, as is often the case with Medicare patients, there are no constraints on their spending. Similarly, if physicians and hospitals are paid to provide these services, there is a clear financial incentive to provide them. Overall, then, both the incentives and constraints are aligned to provide more intrusive and expensive care regardless of the consequences. Also, the fact that such invasive treatments can at best temporarily postpone, but not prevent, death underlines the wasteful futility of this approach.

THE ROLE OF MEDICAL ETHICS IN PERPETUATING THE DEFAULT OPTION

Paradoxically, medical ethicists, who are focused on protecting the safety and dignity of patients, also play an important role in perpetuating the default EOL care model. Under the current code of medical ethics in this country, a patient should be able to make decisions free from coercion and regardless of cost.[14] According to this principle, a patient who chooses to fight to the last breath should not have to face any negative consequences, including the high cost of their care. Conveniently for medical ethicists, very few dying patients in fact have such a concern. That is because the healthcare payment model, driven by insurance reimbursements, financially rewards doctors and hospitals (and, indirectly, patients) that use expensive, high-tech medical devices and procedures to extend life. Nonetheless, as noted by ICU and palliative-care physician Jessica Nutik Zitter in her 2017 book *Extreme Measures*, she and many other doctors believe that respecting patient autonomy should always be an "ethical priority" in providing EOL care.[15] If that means using feeding tubes and a ventilator to keep a dying patient alive well past the point of enjoying life (or even being consciously aware), she nonetheless will honor the patient's request. Chapter 7 will cover the reasoning behind this ethical concept of patient autonomy and suggest an alternative approach.

And so despite the efforts of such caring, conscientious physicians as Dr. Zitter, a natural death advocate, many patients in American healthcare facilities will continue to be caught in the death trap by choice, by ignorance of their options, or, most frequently of all, by default.

TURNING THE TITANIC

In this chapter, I have provided evidence suggesting that the default model for providing EOL care in this country is dysfunctional and in need of urgent reform. However, shifting the current paradigm away from "keeping us alive at all costs" toward an emphasis easing our exit from the world through comfort care will not be easy. As evidenced by the death panels fiasco in 2010—the last time this issue was debated on Capitol Hill—convincing federal lawmakers to pass legislation lowering our likelihood of getting caught in the death trap will be like turning an ocean liner around. The goal is achievable, but it will take aggressive advocacy by reformers and an unprecedented level of cooperation among the major stakeholders in the American healthcare system to make it happen.

If such a change could in fact be brought about—it will not happen overnight (though I should note that I wouldn't have written this book if I didn't believe such change were possible). That does not mean we should be complacent. We can begin by transforming the default care model one individual at a time. We can choose the nature and the limits of the EOL care we wish to receive. Also, we can formalize our wishes in an advance directive and encourage those we care about to do the same.

Through such individual efforts we can save ourselves from the death trap, however, until the U.S. healthcare system reforms its approach to EOL care, far too many people will suffer needlessly.

3

THE FICTION OF LIVING FOREVER

We are not living longer, we are dying longer.

—Lionel Shriver, *Should We Stay or Should We Go: A Novel*

Individually and as a society, we try to convince ourselves that we can avoid growing old and fight succumbing to illness or the breakdown of our physical bodies. Dying, of course, is completely out of the question.

While we may be more guilty of deluding ourselves here in the United States, where youth is both glorified and sought after by many who've left it behind, there is no shortage of death denial elsewhere in the world.

"The brain does not accept that death is related to us," says Israeli neuroscience researcher Dr. Yair Dor-Ziderman, coauthor of a study published in the November 2019 issue of the medical journal *NeuroImage*.[1] "We have this primal mechanism that means when the brain gets information that links self to death, something tells us it's not reliable, so we shouldn't believe it. . . . We cannot rationally deny that we will die, but we think of it more as something that happens to other people."[2]

One way we deal with this unpleasant issue is to institutionalize old age, death, and dying. We do this by placing very old or very sick people in nursing homes or assisted living communities where it is easy to keep them conveniently out of sight and out of mind. In this comforting but illusory world, old age, death, and dying are something that happens to other people—out of sight and out of mind.

Ann Neumann sums up this phenomenon: "We are socialized to believe [death] can somehow be avoided because we don't see it."[3] The absence of death in our daily lives gives us a false sense of security. It tricks us into believing that we can somehow escape this unhappy fate. Moreover, because we refuse to accept our mortality, we do not plan for how we would prefer to die. Thus we unknowingly consign ourselves, at the end of our life, to the agonies of the death trap. When we're caught in it, our final days become a nightmare and not the fairy tale we had longed for. Yet we cling to our childlike fantasies, hoping that old age, infirmity, and death will never catch up with us.

"People don't act or plan appropriately [for end of life]," write Lynda Gratton and Andrew Scott in their 2017 book *The 100-Year Life: Living and Working in an Age of Longevity* "not because they are terrified about the consequences of their actions, but rather because they are . . . [overly] optimistic" about how long they will live and how long they will remain healthy.[4]

What's more, tremendous advances in medical science are feeding our false hope for immortality. These discoveries have changed the way we die today. We live longer but, unfortunately, our extended life often comes with chronic illnesses such as Alzheimer's, cancer, or kidney failure. Curing disease is great throughout much of life, but in old age it may leave us with an existence lacking meaning, purpose, agency, and comfort. Yet many people keep naively hoping science and technology will cure whatever ails them. They embrace the comforting illusion that the increasingly sophisticated (and expensive) medical machines that we have created, such as ventilators, defibrillators, and blood purifiers, can prevent—or postpone—our physical demise. Many people see the modern ICU as a silver bullet that can cure everyone, including patients who are dying. Those unrealistic expectations reveal our collective failure to recognize the curative limits of medicine. They also deny us the option of choosing a natural death over a life artificially extended by machines.

Understanding how to face death is complex intellectually, emotionally, and physically. Diligently pursuing education about what life will be like near the end has been termed by the Lancet Commission "death literacy."[5] Acquiring this knowledge is fundamental to making informed decisions about your healthcare. One particularly useful educational resource in this space is videos. Later in the book, I discuss the research supporting this observation about the effectiveness of videos for EOL care decisions. Two highly recommended videos for better understanding your choices between ICU and comfort care are titled *Extremis* and *End of the Line* both on Netflix.

My bubble of optimism burst at age sixty-four when I underwent quadruple bypass heart surgery. Additionally, I had to have a second round of surgeries to remove the plaque that had built up in both of my carotid arteries. These two critical blood pathways were 100 percent and 80 percent blocked, respectively. Fortunately, these major surgeries were successful, and I received superb medical care. Considering the extent of the blockages in both my heart and my neck, things could have turned out differently. I was fortunate because of these timely interventions to have avoided suffering a heart attack or a stroke.

Following my second carotid artery surgery, my surgeon recommended that I have my carotids checked annually with an ultrasound screening. A year later, I had my first and only ultrasound test. Fortunately, it confirmed that my arteries were free of blockage. I have not had a scan since. Is that irresponsible? I would argue that it is not. Even if I knew my carotids were again filling up with plaque, I would not elect to have this invasive procedure done again. For one thing, it is risky. In addition, it makes no sense to me to keep pursuing medical care that I believe is unlikely to improve my life.

Now in fairness to others, I am not suggesting patients should ignore their physician's advice about receiving routine ultrasound tests. It is a modestly expensive test and one that could very well help identify a correctable problem. However in my particular case, I have concluded that I am old enough to die and not anxious to keep looking for health problems.

The phrase "old enough to die" comes from journalist and political activist Barbara Ehrenreich, author of the 2018 nonfiction book *Natural Causes*.[6] She has a doctorate in biology and a reputation for chronicling cultural shifts before others notice them. In *Natural Causes*, she questions our increasingly unrealistic expectations regarding old age and dying and encourages us to "rethink the prospect of personal control over body and mind."[7]

"We would all like to live longer and healthier lives," she acknowledges, but she then questions "how much of our lives should be devoted to the project."[8] She asserts that like me, she is "no longer interested in looking for [medical] problems that remain undetectable to me."[9]

Like Barbara Ehrenreich, I believe that "being old enough to die is an achievement, not a defect, and the freedom it brings is worth celebrating."[10]

Yet compared to most people, Ms. Ehrenreich and I are in a distinct minority: Only about one in three Americans has prepared an AHD.[11] This is a legally binding document in which an individual may specify the type of medical care they wish to receive at the end of life or, just as importantly, the care they wish *not* to receive.

While it is unclear why so many people have failed to adequately prepare for death, it's logical to conclude that many are clinging—albeit irrationally—to the idea that they will not die or that their death will be swift and peaceful.

Part of this unrealistic attitude toward aging and death stems from our cultural expectations. As a society we are overly optimistic and tend to shun what is likely for what is possible. No one knows when they will die, and many never stop clinging to the idea of immortality. As such, patients keep asking for more treatments even if they are old and frail or fighting a life-threatening illness.

Unfortunately for many of these chronically or acutely ill patients, immortality rarely lives up to its ideal. Take, for example, the nearly 200,000 Medicare-insured patients who are treated each year in long-term-care hospitals (LTCHs) in this country.[12] "Many of [these] people never make it home," writes Dr. Anil Makam, a hospitalist and researcher at the University of California–San Francisco, in an article published in the *Journal of the American Geriatrics Society*.[13] "They go back and forth between the LTCH and [regular] hospitals and nursing facilities, and they die in one of them."[14]

In between their transfers, said Dr. Daniela Lamas, a critical care specialist at Brigham and Women's Hospital in Boston, their existence is far from ideal. "People were bored," she told *New York Times* reporter Paula Span about the fifty LTCH patients she had interviewed for a medical study.[15] "They couldn't move. There was a desperate sense of being alone, feeling trapped."[16]

Yet, noted Dr. Lamas, "most patients expressed optimism about returning to their former lives and hadn't talked to their LTCH doctors about what would happen if they encountered setbacks."[17] Considering their dismal predicament, who could blame these patients for hoping for the best?

The fiction of living forever is a mindset and one that became poignantly clear to me some years ago when I participated in a medical ethics program at the St. Louis University Medical School. At the time I was in my mid-thirties and serving as CEO of St. Joseph Hospital in Chicago. I was the only healthcare executive in my fifteen-member class. Everyone else was either a physician or a medical ethicist. During the two-week program, founded and run by Father Kevin O' Rourke, a Dominican priest and a nationally renowned medical ethicist, we attended morning classes at the medical school. In the afternoon, we sat in on patient case reviews and accompanied hospital physicians on their medical rounds.

On one of those rounds, I met Gerald, a patient at the university hospital. He was a middle-aged alcoholic who needed a liver transplant. His drinking had destroyed his liver. Based on his history of chronic alcohol abuse, the clinical team in charge of his care concluded that he was not a good candidate for a transplant. They knew the probability of Gerald resuming his drinking after he received a new liver was statistically over 90 percent. Consequently the doctors made the difficult decision that should a much sought-after liver become available from an organ donor, they would assign it to a patient who was more likely to survive.

Such trade-offs are required every single day in the medical world. Medicine is not a profession for the faint of heart.

I suggested that the doctors on the clinical team share with Gerald the reasoning behind their decision to deny him a new liver. I figured that since he, in effect, had just been handed a death sentence by them, he had a right to know why. They agreed. They also decided that I would be the best person to have that conversation with the patient.

Though I dreaded my unexpected assignment—which I suspected was my reward for sharing my personal views with these clinicians—I'd known I might face moments like this when I chose a career in healthcare. After taking a few deep breaths to calm myself, I knocked on the door of the doomed patient's room. Gerald greeted me warmly, making me feel even worse than I already did. As we talked, I found Gerald to be a very engaging and likable person. He also was very clever. He told me that if he stood in the clinical team's shoes, he would not give himself the liver.

"Who in their right mind would offer such a rare, life-giving organ to a person with my history?" he said.

But Gerald then emphasized that he was not, in fact, on the clinical team, and if the choice were left up to him, "I would give myself the liver."

Gerald eventually succumbed to his liver disease. Years later I still think of him from time to time, remembering his charm, his humor, and his sad predicament. In medicine, trade-offs are never easy especially when you happen to be the bearer (or the recipient) of bad tidings.

Gerald's story, of course, is hardly unique. We all want to live as long as we can. Nobody wants to be sick or old. Nobody wants to die. This has been true throughout human history. What has changed in modernity is that advancements in medical science now allow doctors to keep us physically alive far longer than ever before. That does not make us immortal, but it does allow us to delude ourselves into thinking that medicine can save us no matter what. While I refer to this mindset as "the fiction of living forever," others call it "delusional optimism" or "willful blindness." Call it what you will, it's what people often, and quite understandably, do to deny death's inevitability. This mindset allows us to postpone the difficult, often painful choices many of us will have to make at the end of our own life or that of a cherished loved one.

The downside of this immortality illusion is that if you are very old or very sick, prolonging your physical life with high-tech medicine does not always translate into a meaningful extension of your life. Life is more than mere existence. You need to ask yourself how postponing your death through medical means will affect the nature of your life during the time you have left. How high a price are you likely to pay for denying yourself the chance to die naturally? How would you respond if you were required to answer this question for someone else? For example, if you were faced with the grave decision of removing life support from a dying loved one, would you see yourself as pulling the plug on his or her life? Or would you see this as a chance to allow your loved one to die naturally?

My siblings and I were suddenly faced with this very difficult choice in February 1990. That is when our seventy-nine-year-old mother, Frances, who, except for brittle bones was in relatively good health, fractured her hip. She unexpectedly sustained this injury just as

I was calling her from my home in Los Altos Hills, California. She was visiting my brother James at his Milwaukee home. When she walked to the telephone that my brother had just answered to speak with me, her hip snapped. She was transported by ambulance to St. Mary's hospital, where my father, Francis Connelly, had worked for thirty years and where I later served on the board of directors.

The bone break was serious enough to require surgery. I immediately made arrangements to fly to Wisconsin, where I spent the next two days at my mother's bedside. She seemed to be recovering well. I flew home, comfortable in the expectation that she was on the mend.

Just after returning to California, however, I received a phone call that is etched in my memory. It was from Sister Renée Rose, a Catholic sister who served as the CEO of St. Mary's Hospital. She also was a close family friend. Sister Renée, who was a Daughter of Charity of St. Vincent de Paul, a Catholic order devoted to helping the needy, informed me that my mother had "thrown an embolism." This means that an air bubble, possibly an unintended artifact of the surgery, had been released into her bloodstream. It had migrated to her brain, causing a massive stroke. She had been transferred to the hospital's ICU, where I was told she was in a persistent vegetative state, meaning she had no detectable brain activity.

All of a sudden, our family was faced with a terrible choice. The doctors caring for my mother saw no practical hope for her recovery. They proposed removing her from life support. This was the woman who had given us life and raised us wisely. My mother was the first person to hold me and love me. Less than a week earlier she'd been in relatively good health. Suddenly she was facing death. My heart was fighting with my mind. Nothing I had experienced during the nearly two decades I had worked in the healthcare field, including helping direct one of the country's first hospices, had prepared me for this moment. I felt as helpless and grief-stricken as anyone else who gets caught up in such a dire predicament.

I thought of asking my mother's doctors to keep her on life support—at least until I could fly back to Milwaukee and say goodbye to her in person. I hoped and prayed for a reversal in her condition, which I knew would require a miracle. I did not want to lose my mother. I did not want to let her go.

I also knew my mother was a brave and sensible person. She had made it clear to my siblings and me that should her life deteriorate to the point that it had lost all joy or meaning, she did not want to stick around. To honor her stated wishes, we removed her from life support.

Had we chosen to prolong her physical existence with ventilators and feeding tubes, we would not have been doing her a favor. She deserved the right to die naturally. Which she did, just one day after throwing the embolism.

My mother did not have an advance directive. She had, however, been very clear with her children that she wanted nothing to do with life-prolonging healthcare. So fortunately for her and us, we knew she did not want her life artificially extended—and we made sure this did not happen. However, learning what to expect at the end of life and spelling out your wishes in an advance directive offer the best way to ensure that you will have the opportunity to die well, as I believe my mother did.

This expression "die well" may seem like an oxymoron—at least until you consider the alternative. If you have any questions about what modern death might entail, visit your local hospital and ask if you can walk through the ICU. Witness the patients hooked up to ventilators, feeding tubes, and dialysis machines. Ask yourself, "Is this how I want to spend my final days? Is this how I want to die?"

If the answer is no and you're getting up there in years like I am, consider educating yourself about your options for EOL care and documenting your preferences in an advance directive. If that is not practical or affordable, you could record your wishes in a cell phone video. Make your family and caregivers aware of your video.

Admittedly, death and dying are not cheerful topics. They are issues that most of us would rather not contemplate. However, taking the trouble to spell out your preferences for EOL medical care is well worth the effort. If nothing else, it might give you peace of mind.

I am not suggesting that I came to my decision easily. As I crafted my approach to how I would use healthcare in old age, I experienced a certain amount of fear and discomfort at the thought of my death. I was forced to relinquish any remaining illusions I might have harbored regarding my own immortality.

Despite the anxiety this stirred up, however, I felt even more fearful of the possibility of someday becoming incompetent and thus losing my ability to make my own care choices at the end of life. I knew from my own long experience working in healthcare that if I had no advance directive, the default healthcare system would step into that vacuum—along with its arsenal of high-tech medical devices and clinical specialists intent on keeping me technically alive even as my body was wasting away.

No one should ever have to die that way. It's misguided and unnecessary, and it consumes limited medical resources. Most importantly, it's inhumane. I wrote this book to give you the tools and knowledge you will need to make sure that you and those you care about do not fall into the death trap and to help you overcome the fear and reluctance everyone naturally feels when planning for EOL care.

4

THE ART AND SCIENCE
OF MEDICINE

Bureaucracy, science, and the law have replaced God and
philosophy as the central organizing forces in our modern
world.

—Alasdair MacIntyre, *After Virtue*

M any people believe that every problem can be solved with science,
including our own mortality. This trend started with the Enlightenment and has advanced further in today's postmodern world. In his
book *The Jefferson Bible*, Peter Manseau describes the influence of the
great philosophers and scientists, including John Locke, Francis Bacon,
and Isaac Newton. "The world was eminently knowable," Manseau
writes, teaching us that we should be "more interested in science than
faith, more in reason than in emotion, more in minute inspection than
intuition or revelation."[1]

This perspective may be erudite, but it is flawed. These presump-
tions have created a global culture in which science is favored over in-
tangibles like wisdom and art. This way of seeing the world is sometimes
codified in a school of thought known as "scientism." It is an excessive
belief in the power of scientific knowledge and techniques. For example,
our collective management of the coronavirus assumed science would pre-
vail. After all, an excessive belief in science gives us the illusion of control.
The truth, however, is that science does not have all the answers. For instance, when it comes to understanding the meaning of life, science cannot
help us. Yet our modern society is uncomfortable with uncertainty or the
fact that science has limits.

Our culture's overreliance on science has profound consequences,
and contrary to popular belief, not all of them are positive. Our rigid de-

pendence on scientific evidence has, at times, come at the cost of losing common sense. Instead of relying on intuition or tradition, we demand pseudoscientific proof for all sorts of subjective decisions. The simple truth is that many decisions have no proof.

Great thinkers from previous generations knew this. Take C. S. Lewis, for instance. While Lewis championed rationality in certain contexts, he also understood that man cannot live by reason and science alone. Indeed, Lewis referred to the "hallowed scientific revolution as a period of 'new ignorance' because he believed that . . . choosing to focus on quantifiable measurement to the exclusion of all other types of inquiry brought modern culture into an ethical and social desert."[2] Referencing common sense today, as a rationale for decisions, is almost *verboten*.

The obsessive focus on quantifiable measurement is evident in modern medicine, and one can't help but agree that this has ushered in an age of new ignorance. Quantification isn't everything—and we must embrace the *qualitative* when facing important decision points in life, like facing death. To quote C. S. Lewis once more: "Human beings spend most of their lives processing the world through *ratio*, reason-using, argument-generating, fact-seeking . . . but in exceptional moments [like facing death] the more elusive, intuitive, contemplative" model may be superior.[3]

SCIENCE DOESN'T EXPLAIN EVERYTHING

The word "placebo" literally means to please or placate. The amazing impact of placebos is that they can relieve pain, diminish symptoms, or enhance healing even though these outcomes are not understood by science. Anne Harrington, a historian of science at Harvard, observed that placebos are "lies that heal."[4]

Thom Krystofiak in his book *Tempted to Believe* uses the concept of placebos to make the point that having religion and faith has benefits even if these beliefs are not provable. Similarly, placebos have benefits that science cannot explain. He observes,

> A placebo reveals, more clearly than anything, that belief itself can
> produce significant positive results, even in the face of a completely

conflicting underlying reality. . . . It is the innate healing capacity of the mind and body, a resource beyond the full understanding of science, which does all the work. . . . You must believe, in essence, that something that is fictitious is real. That is how you get the benefit.[5]

In other words, there are benefits to relying on something other than science to make decisions. Like art, faith and belief offer different approaches to life than science, and they have their own strengths.

SCIENCE AND MEDICINE

Nowhere is the domination of science more evident today than in the practice of medicine. Over the past century, physicians have come to rely almost entirely on science in their approach to care. Traditionally medicine was looked upon as both an art *and* a science.

Historically physicians restored us to health using knowledge and procedures passed down by other practitioners. That model of medical education changed after the famous Flexner Report of 1910.[6] This report required a much more rigorous and scientific approach to medical education. It shifted the focus of medical schools to teaching based almost exclusively on scientific principles. This century-old movement has continued to evolve, and today the major focus of medical schools is on research. The impact of this scientific focus for medical education has been both beneficial and profound. Yet this heavy focus on science and evidence has diminished the role of art in medicine. Until the middle of the last century, it was not uncommon for doctors in this country to forge a personal bond with their patients. Many MDs were general practitioners who would treat and get to know virtually every member of the family. The idealized image of the kind, gentle American family doctor reached its apotheosis in the late 1960s when the hit TV series *Marcus Welby, MD* began airing on ABC. The title character, played by veteran actor Robert Young, used wit and wisdom as well as medical knowledge to save the lives and soothe the agitated spirits of his patients, young and old. He even made house calls! I knew it was time to retire when on making a reference to Dr. Welby in a health-care talk, I discovered that few in my young audience had a clue about Dr. Welby.

Obviously, the old-fashioned style of doctoring once practiced by the Marcus Welbys of America has largely disappeared. Technology today plays the dominant role in the diagnosis and treatment of patients. Instead of spending time getting to know patients, physicians just order tests. It is a sad and significant fact that doctors rarely have the time to get to know their patients. Historically primary care was designed to coordinate a patient's overall care. Today primary care is provided by overworked family practitioners and internists with a large number of patients in their practices. If these physicians encounter a serious medical problem, nine times out of ten they will refer the ailing patient to a specialist. Unfortunately, this model of care means there are multiple physicians caring for a patient, and this has contributed greatly to our system of fragmented care. These physicians seldom talk with each other about their common patients, and that is one reason why healthcare coordination is so poor. There were few specialists in the days of Dr. Welby. Now there are hundreds of new specialties and specialists prepared to treat each unique, diagnosed condition but unable to talk with each other about their patients.

Dr. David Leach has spent his career helping train physicians, including being executive director of the Accreditation Council for Graduate Medical Education (the organization responsible for overseeing the training standards for all medical specialties) for more than a decade. He offers the following perspective on the need to balance art and science.

> Medicine is a craft that uses both science and art. Science generates generalizable and useful facts and principles (guidelines, protocols, etc.); art always deals with the particular. The practical wisdom that is needed in good patient care (*phronesis*) involves both the rules (science) and knowing which rule to break and exactly how far to break it to accommodate the reality of the particular patient (art). It involves a formal act of prudence.[7]

Unfortunately in our science-obsessed society, the virtues of prudence are often ignored. Don't get me wrong. The shift toward specialization and science in medicine has brought undeniable benefits such as the miracle drugs and sophisticated treatments we have developed for diagnosing and curing the sick and the injured. However there is also a downside, particularly when it comes to providing artful and compassionate EOL care. Too often we try to keep dying patients physically alive by using advanced medical techniques despite the impossibility of their ultimate recovery. Instead of calling on science to artificially extend their lives, we should be using our basic human decency and common sense—the artful side of medicine—to help them die naturally.

Professor Charles C. Camosy of Fordham University argues that modern medicine has become secularized, undermining our fundamental sense of humanity. He observes, "Contemporary medicine is often geared toward avoiding or forestalling death—which is at odds with a religious approach that emphasizes the reality of death and highlights the limitations of medicine to avoid or forestall it."[8]

One example of how medicine and society secularize death is the legal definition of death itself. The definition is purely clinical. This clinical definition itself is controversial among clinicians. But the definition excludes considerations of one's faith and how that faith might impact their perception of death. Camosy pointedly expresses his concern: "Medical science and tests can be used to determine whether death has taken place, but deciding what death is in the first place can be determined only by asking theological questions."[9]

The key point is that for individuals of faith, dying isn't just a clinical or legal issue.

As a society we invest generously in medical technology, yet we are unwilling to fund critical, non-medical support, like homecare, which is especially important for the frail and elderly. We also fall woefully short in providing palliative and hospice care to terminal patients who would prefer to die at home rather than in a hospital.

By relying almost exclusively on procedures and tests and particularly in our treatment of dying patients, we are taking not just the art but also the humanity out of medicine. Our strictly scientific approach focuses primarily on clinical rather than spiritual and psychological considerations such as the emotional well-being of the patient. Arguably these less-tangible factors are just as important, if not more important, than science in delivering the comfort and healing that have defined the physician's role since Hippocrates—known as the Father of Medicine—established the ethical foundation of modern medicine in the fifth century BC.

The Hippocratic approach to medicine called on physicians to be "very kind to the patient." The approach specified gentle treatment and "emphasized keeping the patient clean and sterile."[10] This kinder, gentler approach to medicine, employing empathy and intuition, is especially important in treating patients in the last years of their life. By connecting personally with their patients and granting them the dignity and respect that they deserve, doctors can do more to ease their dread and discomfort than any inanimate machine no matter how sophisticated or efficient it may be. Indeed, it is apparent that the more machines dying patients are hooked up to, the lonelier, more hopeless, and more isolated they are likely to feel in their final hours and days. In too many U.S. hospital units today, science prevails over art in EOL care. However it is a Pyrrhic victory, benefiting no one.

I am not alone in questioning both the ethics and practicality of scientism particularly as it relates to medicine. In an article published in *Medium Daily Digest*, Danish data scientist Jonatan Pallesen asserts that contemporary society's overemphasis on solving every problem scientifically is causing significant harm. While acknowledging that science "has prevented and eradicated disease, and brought prosperity to the world like few other things," Pallesen also posits that

> scientism is an underrated problem in the modern world, causing a large amount of damage. One good . . . example of this is the 1992 official food pyramid (promulgated by the U.S. Department of Agriculture). Just look at how ridiculous that thing is. And it was presented to the public as scientific truth, likely causing millions of people to change their diet for the worse.[11]

This food pyramid promoted a low-fat diet without distinguishing between good fat and bad fat. Consequently, fat in food was replaced by sugar. The result of this scientific advice was more obesity and more diabetes for our nation.

One need not be a research scientist to realize that we need to restore the balance between art and science in medicine. To give just one example of how these two essential healthcare components could work successfully in tandem, we could artfully use data that is scientifically generated to more accurately measure the likelihood of complications arising from specific treatment approaches for illnesses that plague the elderly. By sharing the findings of such studies with older patients, we could help them make more informed choices about their EOL care.

Louise Aronson, a 2020 Pulitzer Prize finalist, university professor, and geriatrician, argues that medical science alone is too crude a tool for treating older patients. "Science prioritizes what's easy to measure rather than what matters [to these patients]," she writes in *Elderhood*.[12] She uses the example of a heart attack, in which "we look at outcomes such as time from hospital arrival to catheter treatment, use of medications, and mortality. But the heart attack of an eighty-year-old with a seventeen-item problem list differs from the heart attack of an otherwise healthy fifty-five-year-old who collapses while jogging even if the same heart vessel is clogged to the same degree at the same place."[13]

Standard medical measures such as these "leave out outcomes of critical importance to older patients, such as return to prior cognitive function, loss of key abilities and independence, [and] risk of nursing home placement," says Dr. Aronson.[14]

For her own part, whenever Dr. Aronson assesses a new patient, she doesn't rely on dry, one-size-fits-all medical statistics. What matters to her most as a physician is finding out "who a person is and where they are in [their] life."[15]

In deciding on a treatment regimen, she doesn't ignore science but neither does she allow technical minutiae to color her view of the patient. Like Hippocrates, she understands that forging a bond of trust and understanding with the patient is essential if she hopes to provide them with quality medical care.

As a recent example, the COVID pandemic revealed an overreliance on science in the care of the dying. How our society treated the elderly dying in hospitals and nursing homes during this pandemic is an example of how the healthcare system can devalue common sense and compassion. Thousands of elderly were forced to die alone in institutions without family by their side. The fear of spreading COVID was the sole factor considered in allowing people to die this way. The federal government, through Medicare, initiated this policy. Federal mandates meant that these institutions could not have visitors. Why weren't families allowed to bring family members home so those family members could be close to their loved ones as they were dying? Why weren't these patients given the option of hospice at home?

Because we wouldn't accept the risks. Statistically speaking, these COVID risks may have been a reasonable trade-off for many. Families, if given the choice, may well have been willing to assume the risk and allow themselves to be with their dying loved ones. Knowing when to offer this choice is the art of medicine, and it requires prudence.

HUMANITIES AS A THERAPEUTIC TREATMENT

What can help prepare us to leave the material world? Being ready to let go is a part of the dying process. Do we have to choke ourselves to death with technology before we learn how to do it? Perhaps we should instead turn to our senses for therapeutic treatment. Neither science nor art alone can help us understand the dying process. Through the synthesis of science and art we are more likely to find a good death. What might the therapeutic art of medicine look like in the dying process? It begins with helping the individual make sense out of their life. It requires learning how to conceptualize letting go of life—your life. These are philosophical reflections that have clinical implications. When to let go is a decision only you can make.

Some may choose to fight death, to never give up. However, we all must accept that death will come. The real question is how do we wish to face death? This is a humanitarian (art) question more than a scientific one.

One philosophical theory that can help is the concept of detachment. Aging is full of these gradual detachments. We lose our energy, we lose our endurance (two big losses for me), we lose our strength, we lose our youthful bodies, we lose our mental capabilities, and eventually we lose our independence. These are painful losses. Some of us experience these losses more intensely than others. All of these losses perhaps are preparation for the ultimate letting go— detaching ourselves from life itself, knowing our life was meaningful and had great purpose but also accepting that the world will go on quite well without us. Detachment requires humility.

Our cultural bias toward science has deprioritized the hospice care option. Selecting hospice means the patient or their representative is letting go of further medical treatments. Hospice is a humanitarian model not a science-based model. Going into hospice is giving up on scientific cures. Neither physicians, patients, nor families want to make this choice—to let go. Ironically there is scientific evidence that has helped popularize hospice: research has documented that life expectancy is just as long, if not longer, in hospice care. This research reminds me of a rather blunt quote from a physician advising her patient about a chemotherapy regime: "You probably have six months left to live. You can take chemotherapy and you will suffer through those six months, or you can go into hospice and spend that time putting your affairs together with your family."

Such humanitarian advice is rare in healthcare, but it may be prudent. The point here is that death involves making complicated personal and clinical choices. Do we want chemotherapy, or do we want hospice? Such dilemmas would benefit from a therapeutic perspective and humanitarian reflection.

DEATH IS A CONUNDRUM

Some EOL issues defy easy categorization. They are neither art nor science. Instead they seem to emerge from an elusive realm that one might encounter in an episode of *The Twilight Zone*.

Meet Mary Flanagan, a patient at Chicago's St. Joseph Hospital where I was CEO. In 1983, this retired, sixty-eight-year-old, Chicago public grade-school teacher was admitted to the hospital following a massive heart attack. In the vast majority of such cases, the patient dies. In this case, St. Joseph's highly skilled medical professionals were able to save her. Unfortunately they could not undo the irreparable brain damage she had suffered before her arrival at the ER. She had stopped breathing for a prolonged period of time, depriving her brain of oxygen. As result, Mary Flanagan had entered a persistent vegetative state. Aided by a ventilator, she continued breathing, but the vibrant, former pedagogue beloved by generations of Chicago youngsters was gone. The brain damage she had suffered could not be reversed. The doctors told her family the breathing machine and the feeding tube they had surgically inserted into Mary Flanagan's body were the only things standing between her and the grave.

The family took the news with difficulty, but they would not give up on her. Since Mary had no AHD, they would have to determine her fate. They decided to keep her going as long as possible regardless of the quality of her existence. Mary's husband, James, visited her faithfully almost every day.

Six months after she was admitted to St. Joseph's, Mary's Blue Cross and Medicare hospital insurance policies had both reached their limits. Normally in such a situation the hospital would have discharged her to a ventilator-qualified nursing home. However, the hospital worked with the family to qualify Mary for Medicaid. Although the insurance payments fell far short of covering the actual costs incurred by St. Joseph's in caring for Mary (the shortfall was around $300 a day), I worked with our social work and billing departments to find ways to help her stay. The family had seen how lovingly the nursing team had cared for Mary—she never had a single bedsore—and they desperately wanted her to be able to remain in their care.

Around this same time, I arranged for a priest from the hospital's pastoral care department to meet with Mary's family to discuss the possibility of taking her off the ventilator. As a fellow Catholic I understood their feelings about the sacredness of life. But as a health-care professional I also knew that keeping Mary alive artificially was, at best, an exercise in futility. For her sake and theirs, I wanted to help them let her go.

The priest told James Flanagan and Mary's other close family members that turning off the breathing machine would be an act of mercy and thus would not violate church doctrine. By removing her from the ventilator, he advised, they would not be killing her. They would be allowing her to go to her heavenly reward in a peaceful, dignified way.

After mulling over the priest's counsel for several days, James Flanagan informed us that the family decided to keep Mary on the ventilator.

Did the family members make their decision based on their religious beliefs? Did they think they were doing the right thing for their loved one? Or did they simply want to avoid taking responsibility for ending Mary's life, possibly the most difficult decision any family can ever be asked to make? Did they expect Mary would someday walk out of the hospital under her own power? If so, they were deluding themselves. But who has the right to criticize someone for hoping for a miracle? As stated earlier in this book, when my own mother became brain dead in 1990, my siblings and I faced the same agonizing choice the Flanagans were forced to make six years earlier. In retrospect, I know how confused and upset they must have felt.

Unfortunately, James Flanagan also was in fragile health when his wife fell gravely ill. He passed away about two years into Mary's hospitalization.

Following his death, Mary's niece Grace kept up the family's hospital vigil. She visited her stricken aunt weekly. Just as James Flanagan had done before her, every time she sat by Mary's bedside, Grace spoke to her. Neither she nor her late uncle knew if she could hear them. Nonetheless, they somehow felt they needed to have these conversations with her.

After underwriting Mary's care at the hospital for two years, Medicaid decided that for economic reasons she needed to be moved to a less expensive medical facility that specialized in ventilator patients. Though upset by this decision, the family, which was of modest means, had no choice but to comply. The night before Mary was to be transferred to the specialized nursing home, Grace once again visited her aunt. Though Mary had never visibly responded to anything she said, she decided to tell her about the impending move.

On the following morning when the nurses came into Mary's hospital room to start preparing her for the transfer, they discovered she had died during the night.

The family deemed the timing of Mary's passing a miracle. They took it as a sign that all those years of visiting and talking to her had not been in vain. Despite what the doctors had told them about Mary's unresponsive medical state, they concluded that Mary had in fact been able to hear them. They believed she did not want to leave the hospital at which she was receiving saint-like care and that God had granted her wish to die.

If I were more cynical, I might conclude that this was a convenient way for the family to justify putting Mary Flanagan through almost three years of misery that she need not have endured. But I too believe that divine intervention is possible. Indeed, it is difficult to imagine that something supernatural was *not* at work at St. Joseph Hospital when you consider the fact that a patient who had clung fiercely to life for three long years suddenly died at the very moment her insufferable situation threatened to get even worse.

Who is to say that Mary Flanagan was not listening to her loved ones chattering away at her bedside? Stranger things have happened— and not just at St. Joseph Hospital. I have witnessed similarly mysterious events at other healthcare facilities where I have worked. Sadly, not all of those patients' stories had salvational endings. I would like to have seen more of them turn out the way Mary Flanagan's did.

There are aspects of dying that are mysterious. Science should not be the only guide we use on our journey in the final stage of life. One of America's most influential philosophers eloquently offers this wisdom: "There is a chasm between knowledge and ignorance which the arches of science can never span."[16]

5

THE ETHICS AND ECONOMICS OF
END-OF-LIFE CARE

> No generation can contract debts greater than can be paid
> during the course of its existence. . . . We must not let our
> rulers load us with perpetual debt.
>
> —Thomas Jefferson

If the Founding Fathers were alive today, they would be appalled at how deeply the United States has buried itself in debt. Long before the COVID-19 crisis of 2020 sparked trillions of dollars in emergency spending, the United States already faced a multi-trillion-dollar deficit, much of it due to spending on federal entitlement programs such as Social Security, Medicare, and Medicaid. Our national debt in 2008 was $10 trillion.[1] By 2016, that debt had doubled to $20 trillion.[2] Even more disturbing than the national debt is the specter of unfunded liabilities—promises made by our government to us—that now stand at $101 trillion for Social Security and Medicare alone.[3] Some estimates range as high as $210 trillion when all unfunded liabilities are taken into account (including items like student debt and Fannie Mae). Perhaps most frightening are two statistics: (1) 37 percent of *all U.S. dollars* were created over the eighteen months between 2020 and the first six months of 2021; and (2) national debt is roughly three times the size of the entire U.S. economy.[4] This level of debt is unsustainable and will result in serious adverse consequences in the not-too-distant future.

Certainly we are a healthier and more just society today because of these social-safety-net programs, which provide financial and healthcare assistance to some of America's most vulnerable citizens. The only problem is the funds in the U.S. treasury are not infinite and the way in which we currently distribute this federal largesse is out of balance.

According to the Congressional Budget Office (CBO), in 1960 the federal government spent 52 percent of its annual budget on programs that benefited the young such as Aid to Dependent Children and the National School Lunch Program.[56] Just 11 percent of federal funds went to programs for the elderly. Five years later, that ratio began to shift with the enactment of Medicare and Medicaid. Fast forward more than half a century to 2017. By that year, says the CBO, the spending ratio of 1960 had completely reversed itself: 45 percent of our federal dollars were spent on the elderly while children's programs received just 9 percent of the national budget.[7]

Looked at from a purely economic point of view, the United States has become a gerontocracy, a society that supports its senior citizens first then looks toward the welfare of its children almost as an afterthought.

As a senior citizen, I benefit from this funding imbalance. I am covered by highly affordable Medicare health insurance, and I receive a Social Security payment every month. Naturally I am grateful for these benefits and believe that the government is doing the right thing by supporting the elderly. On the other hand, favoring seniors over youth in our federal spending is immoral and needs to change. It may be a cliche, but our children *are* the country's future. We have an obligation to look after their welfare which is at least as compelling as the welfare of the elderly.

If we were to spend more to ensure the health, education, and economic security of our children, we would not be setting any kind of precedent. Every other industrialized democracy on earth spends proportionately more on their children than we do.

According to Brookings Institution economist Louise Sheiner, however, we can neither direct more federal funding to our children nor sustain our increasingly expensive programs for the elderly unless we do two very unpopular things: raise federal income taxes and reduce spending on Medicare and Social Security. "Our [national] debt path is unsustainable," asserts Sheiner, and it will remain so, unless we undertake these "significant changes."[8]

I agree with both conclusions of this distinguished economist, who is the policy director of the Hutchins Center on Fiscal and Monetary

Policy and a former senior economist for the Council of Economic Advisers. We need to raise tax revenue to meet our fiscal obligations, and we need to reduce federal spending, particularly on healthcare. The United States spends more than double the amount that other advanced nations spent per capita on healthcare. Yet ironically, these other nations often have better patient outcomes. Notably, these countries provide patients much better access to less expensive primary care and homecare but less access to high-tech care than we do.

These fundamental differences in treatment approaches, patient outcomes, and healthcare spending are most telling in our very different approaches to EOL care. As noted earlier, when tending to a dying patient, U.S. doctors often extend the dying process through high-tech gadgetry. It is easier to get a transplant consultation than it is to have a palliative consultation. By using expensive, sophisticated machines, they may keep the patient breathing for a few more weeks or months, in some cases with negative results. In too many instances, patients receive high-tech care like a hospital ICU when they really need hospice.

Let's look at the financial side of the problem. In 2019, Medicare spending topped $650 billion.[9] According to healthcare researchers, a significant portion of this expenditure was on EOL care.[10] In a study of Medicare beneficiaries published in the March 2019 issue of the *American Journal of Hospice and Palliative Medicine*, Doctors Ian Duncan, Tamin Ahmed, Henry Dove, and Terri Maxwell found that depending on who was providing the data, in calendar year 2015 spending on Medicare beneficiaries in the last year of life ranged from 13 percent to 25 percent of the beneficiary's lifetime Medicare spending.[11] They concluded that the higher estimates "more accurately reflect the full cost of a patient's last year of life."[12] Notably, they also found that "more effective use of palliative care and hospice benefits offers a lower cost, higher quality alternative [to curative care] for patients at end of life."[13]

Their statistical finding that about one-quarter of Medicare spending supports patients in the last year of life is consistent with other studies. For example, this matches the results of a long-term study of EOL care spending patterns by Medicare beneficiaries published in the April 2010 issue of *Health Services Research*. In what may be the most comprehensive study of EOL care spending ever undertaken, Centers for Medicare and Medicaid Services staff researchers Gerald Riley and James Lutz found a slight decline in the share of Medicare payments going to persons in the last year of life—from 28.3 percent in 1978 to 25.1 percent in 2006.[14] However they also concluded that this percentage "did not change significantly between 1978 and 2006."[15]

The authors noted that the spending ratio had remained steady despite the fact that "medical technology has changed dramatically over the 29 years of the study and despite increases in both aggressive and nonaggressive care at the end of life among the elderly."[16] They also concluded that "the substantial growth in hospice payments," which Medicare began reimbursing in 1983, "indicates that palliative and supportive care is becoming more common" at the end of life.[17] It is not common enough, however, to change the spending pattern. Because of the rapidly growing number of Medicare beneficiaries in this country, healthcare spending at the end of life continues to rise every year.

There have also been studies challenging the magnitude of EOL care spending. One of the more impressive studies comes from faculty at MIT, Harvard, and Stanford in *Science*. This study acknowledges the commonly cited statistic that 25 percent of life spending for Medicare patients occurs in the last year of life.[18] This study, however, challenges that assumption based on an argument that death is highly unpredictable. Based on their analysis using predictive modeling of death, they argue only 5 percent of Medicare spending is consumed by patients in their last year of life. They justify this position by ignoring the nature of one's existence in the last year of life. Suffice it to say there may be legitimate conflict on exactly how much is spent at the end of life. But there is really no controversy that it is a tremendous amount of money and that this money is poorly spent.

When discussing EOL care costs in this country, it is impor-tant to keep in mind that all financial roads lead to Medicare. The reimbursement rates set by America's largest health insurer set the economic standard by which private insurers base their rates. Right now, Medicare policies and reimbursement rates favor curative care over comfort care. For example, Medicare more than adequately funds surgery but not palliative care. As a result, there are a plethora of surgeons available to perform expensive procedures on dying patients but very few palliative-care physicians to ease their exit from the world. Doctors choose to become surgeons in part because these medical specialists earn a very good living. If Medicare were to change its reimbursement policies to pay gerontologists and palliative-care physicians closer to the amount we now pay surgeons and other highly skilled medical specialists, this would bring about a fundamental shift in the economics of EOL care.

Such a major change to the reimbursement model obviously would not be easily embraced by the status quo. Eventually, however, it could incentivize more young doctors to specialize in geriatrics, palliative care, and primary care because they would now be able to make a good living in specialties that have been ignored and underpaid for years. From my perspective, this underpayment has come at a significant cost to society.

Changing financial incentives is the key to reforming EOL care. The changes would need to be implemented on both an individual and a system-wide basis. We could incentivize Medicare beneficiaries, for instance, to plan for their EOL care by requiring them to complete an AHD and a healthcare power of attorney (HCPA) when they first enroll in Medicare. We could reward enrollees who completed video courses on EOL issues by discounting their Medicare fees. (This proposal is discussed in more detail in chapter 13.)

Numerous studies have shown that an informed patient generally prefers comfort care to curative care once they truly understand their options.[19] In addition, surveys show that most doctors avoid high-tech curative approaches for *their* EOL care.[20] Physicians are perhaps the most informed patients, and they choose comfort care most often. Learning this was one of the reasons I chose comfort care for myself and spelled out my preference in an AHD.

Admittedly, getting the U.S. Congress to approve such an important Medicare reform without sparking a new death-panel debate in which legislators who support EOL planning are demonized for their views would be challenging. But this would be child's play compared to reforming the current healthcare payment model, which financially incentivizes surgery and other expensive medical interventions at the end of life that cost hundreds of millions of dollars a year. We could reverse this dynamic by incentivizing less costly but often more humane and effective treatment approaches such as palliative care and hospice care.

In 2015, the Institute of Medicine (IOM) issued a national set of recommendations titled "Dying in America—Improving Care at End of

Life and Honoring Individual Preferences Near the End of Life. This substantial report was intended to reinforce and strengthen previous reports from the IOM in 1997 and 2003 titled "Approaching Death: Improving Care at the End of Life." These recommendations offered an excellent path for improving EOL care. However virtually none of these wise recommendations have seen the light of day. Let me quote just one conclusion from the last IOM study (which is 612 pages).

> In the end of life arena, there are opportunities for savings by avoiding acute care services that patients and families do not want and are unlikely to benefit them. The Committee that produced this report believes these savings would free up funding for relevant services . . . that would ensure a better quality of life for people near the end of life and protect and support their families.[21]

This quote succinctly describes a key reason for my writing this book. The wise recommendations from these studies—now almost a decade old—remain on the bookshelf. These recommendations deserve to be implemented. The reason these recommendations are not heeded is explained by basic economics. We need to reward the behavior we want. But physicians and patients have very few economic rewards or clinical motivations for following the IOM recommendations. If we want to reform EOL care, we need to start with reforming the payment system. (Chapters 12 and 13 describe specific payment model reforms.)

No one can predict what federal lawmakers will do if and when this Medicare reform is officially proposed. What is clear is that beneficiaries, their families, and the economy all would benefit from a shift toward comfort care at the end of life.

Until Medicare spending is curtailed, a disproportionate amount of our healthcare dollars will go to seniors, and as noted previously, a significant amount of that spending will take place in the last year of life. Moreover the level of spending on older Americans will soar as our population continues to age. The number of Americans over sixty-five is expected to increase dramatically over the next ten years from 54 million in 2017 to 80 million in 2030.[22] The CBO estimates that the bill for medical services for this burgeoning army of seniors will rise by 60 percent during that same decade.[23] Who is going to pay for this? The answer is the same as it was in 1935 when Congress first approved

President Franklin Roosevelt's groundbreaking Social Security Act and in 1965 when President Lyndon Johnson got Medicare and Medicaid enacted: younger wage earners through their payroll taxes.

Today, however, due to America's plunging birthrate and this increase in the number of senior citizens, the funding mechanism is breaking down. According to an April 2019 report by CBS News, Medicare will "become insolvent by 2026 if no changes are made to payroll taxes or how health providers are paid."[24]

Not only is the funding mechanism breaking down but the needs and demands of the elderly are projected to grow tremendously. According to Dr. Joanne Lynn, a national policy expert on public health and geriatrics, growing chronic illness and our aging population are creating a class of "disabled frail elderly."[25] She defines disabled frail elderly as requiring help with daily living (e.g., walking, cooking, shopping, bathing). She estimates that 20 percent of the elderly will experience 5 years of this existence. She indicates the average period of being disabled and frail will be two years. Finally, she estimates that in the next fifteen years this population will double.

According to Lionel Shriver, author of the dystopian novel *The Mandibles: A Family, 2029–2047*, the financial train wreck awaiting us just down the road was largely created by members of America's Baby Boom generation, of which I am a member.[26] While pursuing our right to Social Security income and Medicare benefits, Shriver argues, we have not considered the onerous financial impact of these payments on the next generation. Unless we Boomers start taking our responsibility for draining the U.S. treasury as seriously as we take our rights, says Shriver, we could bankrupt America.

This award-winning American novelist and journalist is correct. But Boomers are not the only culprits in this disaster scenario. Everyone in America is incentivized by the current healthcare system to consume healthcare services. Millions of us get healthcare insurance well below its cost through our employer or the federal government with Medicare and Medicaid. As a result we often consume healthcare services without thinking about their actual cost, which is far more than we are required to pay.

One practical step we could take collectively to contribute to solving this problem would be to voluntarily stop overconsuming healthcare services. By this I am suggesting we begin by viewing healthcare as a resource that needs to be conserved. Adopting this conservation model will require a fundamental attitudinal shift on the part of healthcare consumers, and particularly senior citizens, who are responsible for a disproportionate amount of that spending. My fellow seniors and I will have to stop running to a doctor every time we have a minor complaint or stop trying to screen themselves for a growing list of illnesses. This may sound harsh, but we must learn to live with the chronic illnesses that bedevil almost all of us as we age. I'm not saying, "Stop taking your medicine" or "Don't consult a physician if you're experiencing chest pain." I am saying that the future of healthcare spending in this country is in all of our hands, and each of us can help reduce it by the decisions we make every day.

One rather provocative but interesting idea for changing the economic incentives driving EOL care was debated by two prominent U.S. physicians and a healthcare economist during an August 2017 podcast titled "The Glorious Sunset." The participants were asked to address a proposal made by Tim Price, chief investment officer for a public pension fund. He proposed that health insurance companies offer financial incentives to terminal patients who are willing to forgo standard (curative) EOL medical care.

"When a patient receives a terminal diagnosis," Mr. Price argued, "I have to believe that the healthcare [insurance] companies have actuaries and data sets that would give guidance on what the next six to twenty-four months of medical care would cost." For the patients willing to skip this type of care, the idea being proposed is for a bonus of approximately 50 percent of the difference between the projected cost of standard (curative) medical care and the estimated cost of hospice or palliative care, which is always lower. Under such an arrangement, Mr. Price asserted, both the patient and the health insurer would benefit financially.[27]

One of the debaters, Dr. Ezekiel Emanuel, who chairs the Department of Medical Ethics and Health Policy at the University of Pennsylvania, said he likes the idea of giving patients a choice of the type of care they will receive. But he doesn't like the proposal's emphasis on saving money.

"We should really focus on patients and families and try to make this traumatic event [dying] as smooth and comforting as possible," suggested this medical ethicist. "And we haven't got it right, we sort of pound on [terminal patients'] chests and try to resuscitate them even when that may not be what they want. And I think trying to get patients what they want ought to be our primary focus."[28]

Another debater, the late Professor Uwe Reinhardt of Princeton University, who was one of the world's leading health economists, suggested that some patients might reject the proposed cash offer because it would take away the medical care promised to them by their medical insurer.

"If you have essentially bought and paid for that coverage, for all that end-of-life care, through your insurance," he asked rhetorically, "aren't you entitled to something?"[29]

Reinhardt also opined that private health insurers would not like the idea because in the long run, they would benefit more financially by maintaining the status quo.

> As an insurer, you are just passing through [passing on] hospital and doctor bills and you get little margin [profit] on them—usually around 3 to 5 percent. So your incentive is, in many ways, to increase health spending because then you'll get 3 percent on a higher output [a higher amount of employer health spending], which is why these guys [private health insurers] traditionally have never regulated or controlled costs at all.[30]

The third debate participant, Dr. Thomas Smith, an oncologist and professor of oncology and palliative medicine at Johns Hopkins University Medical School, asserted that "trying to do what is being proposed would be very difficult."[31]

In effect, said Dr. Smith, the health insurer would be asking the ailing patient to give up some of his or her remaining time on earth in exchange for cash. He believes patients faced with such an existential dilemma would find it "too hard to choose."[32]

Overall these unorthodox proposals are meant to stimulate creative thinking rather than propose solutions to reduce our spending on healthcare at the end of life.

The American healthcare system is geared toward providing expensive, high-tech cures and keeping people alive at any cost. It takes courage and resolve to go against the system. The upside is that the benefits of preventing your own or a loved one's needless suffering at the end of life can be immeasurable.

A superb example of how out of balance the current health system is when treating the elderly was published in the January 2020 issue of the *Atlantic Monthly*. It was written by Dr. Ezekiel Emanuel, one of the physicians who participated in the podcast debate discussed above. He reveals how wrong things can go when the medical system goes into its default mode—in this case, in response to a medical crisis experienced by his frail ninety-two-year-old father. His father lived in Chicago and was taken by ambulance to a local hospital ER because he could not get up from a fall. He received a computed tomography (CT) scan, which identified a tumor the size of a pear in his brain. He was immediately hospitalized, and the health system kicked into high gear to cure him. Dr. Emanuel immediately flew to Chicago to help handle the situation, which as an experienced physician he quickly realized was grave.

"My father had a large brain tumor that could not be cured," Emanuel wrote. "No neurosurgeon or oncologist could change the inevitable."[33]

Yet the hospital had already brought in a neurosurgeon and neuro-oncologist to discuss treatment options. None of the attending physicians asked either the patient or his son if the elder Emanuel had an AHD. If the doctors had inquired, they would have learned that the AHD clearly stated the father's desire to avoid major surgery at the end of life. It also articulated a strong preference to die at home.

In addition to correcting this critical oversight by the hospital staff, Dr. Emanuel requested a palliative-care consult and homecare assistance. He was informed that those services were not easily available. Yet his father had already been given intravenous fluids, oxygen, and antibiotics, none of which was needed. He also had been scheduled for various tests to prepare for surgery. After freeing his father from the death trap of an artificially extended life that would have needlessly increased his suffering, Dr. Emanuel took his father home. As a result, he was able to die naturally, surrounded by his family, knowing that his wishes were being honored.

"We still don't have all the bills," wrote Dr. Emanuel, spotlighting another unfortunate aspect of the death trap: the enormous waste of financial resources on expensive, high-tech, unnecessary, and ultimately futile medical procedures.[34] "But the tab for just 12 hours in the hospital came to $19,276.83. In contrast, the more than 200 hours of home care my father got over the next 10 days cost only $6,093."[35]

Unfortunately not every vulnerable patient has someone like Dr. Emanuel in his corner. I would like to see our system changed so that the default EOL care model does not kick in automatically at the end of life, wasting billions of dollars that could be put to better use by society and causing unnecessary suffering for patients.

6

THE PHYSICIAN'S BURDEN

Most doctors are prisoners of their education and shackled by their profession.

—Richard Diaz

CHAOS IN THE PHYSICIAN-PATIENT RELATIONSHIP

A strong physician-patient relationship is essential to providing effective medical care. Without this relationship, neither the patient nor the physician can truly understand each other's point of view, and such mutual misunderstanding can lead to disaster. And while it has evolved over the years, today the physician-patient relationship is generally on shaky ground.

Historically, this relationship was one-sided, and the physician decided what was best for the patient. Understandably, there were flaws with that approach and it needed to change. The next stage in this relationship went in the other direction by emphasizing the patient's power of autonomy. While well intentioned, the patient autonomy approach is also flawed. Letting patients determine by themselves their care creates a new set of problems. The physician is not merely a technician nor a passive observer.

Physicians have ethical obligations to their profession. They have the right to refuse to provide the care they believe would be harmful or futile; they have an ethical obligation to avoid prescribing addictive pharmaceuticals—even when the consumer-oriented patient demands them.

These physician obligations can run counter to the patient's wishes, resulting in friction between the two. As is the case in many areas of life, the goal is to find a suitable middle ground. To quote Dr. Mark Seigler of the University of Chicago, we must balance "the rights of patients and the responsibilities of patients—and the rights of physicians and the responsibilities of patients—at a time when societal values and expectations are changing. This is the critical challenge facing medicine" (Searching for Moral Certainty in Medicine, New York Academy of Medicine, April 24, 1980, Dr. Mark Seigler, University of Chicago, Pritzker School of Medicine).

In addition to this balancing act, there is another variable to consider: the fact that patient care today involves multiple physician-patient relationships. This matrix of relationships further complicates the situation and is one of the key drivers of fragmented healthcare in America.

Fortunately, there is a solution—physicians actually speaking with their patients. Coordinating care is challenging enough with the coding system for physician billing, which effectively eliminates any time for meaningful conversation. As we all know, developing a functional relationship, not to mention establishing mutual expectations, takes time. That is why we must move away from an emphasis on the coding system, and instead embrace a holistic coordination of care.

The physician-patient relationship is especially important in EOL. Understanding how a patient wants to use healthcare in their last few years requires regular conversations. The truth is that many physicians would rather not discuss death with a patient. It's convenient enough for them to avoid these tough conversations since they are not adequately compensated for this effort. Not to mention the fact that a physician's true obligations in this domain are ambiguous at best in today's healthcare system.

All of that said, these concerns are even more critical in EOL care.

Physicians understand perhaps better than anyone else that death is inevitable. It is a natural and inescapable part of life. On a personal level, however, more than one of my doctor friends has confided in me that losing a patient, even an elderly or terminally ill one, can make them feel they have, as one of them put it, "lost the battle against death." They sometimes ask themselves, "What could I have done differently that might have kept this person alive?"

Looking at the issue from an outsider's perspective and without the grave responsibility of holding a human life in my hands, I would respectfully suggest that a more relevant question might be "What can I do to ease this person's passing to the other side?"

In fact, when caring for a terminal patient, most physicians and nurses who work alongside them would prefer to do everything in their power to make the dying process as painless and trauma free as possible. Rendering such tender mercies to their patients at the end of life is just one of many reasons I hold healers in such high esteem.

Dr. Daniela J. Lamas, a *New York Times* writer and critical care physician at Brigham and Women's Hospital in Boston, discusses her struggles with EOL care in an ICU, noting there comes a point for many patients when there is nothing more that can be done.

> Struggling to come to terms with this reality . . . [families often beg us] to continue our interventions . . . [to give them more time to accept this reality]. So we keep [the patient] intubated, deeply sedated and we hope, pain-free, performing the rituals until the family is ready to say good-bye. There is a largely unacknowledged moment in critical care when doctors and nurses shift from caring from the patient in front of us to caring for their loved ones.[1]

These routine occurrences are certainly an understandable reaction by grieving families. But are they fair to the patient, the medical team, and society?

This is just one example of how doctors are pressured to extend a patient's life beyond the point of reasonableness. Let me share an even more emotionally tense example of physicians' environmental pressures in modern medicine.

Ben, a superb cardiologist and long-time friend who has been practicing in a large midwestern city for the past thirty years, asked his colleagues whether they fear family retaliation if they do not over-treat dying patients. "All the physicians I spoke to clearly agreed that the veiled threat of dissatisfaction with care [leading to lawsuits] was present in many cases, which influenced the doctors to provide additional care or prolong resuscitation efforts with little or no chance of success."

"Unwelcome and unfair pressures are placed on a treating physician by both colleagues and families on a regular basis." He added, chillingly,

"A lifelong adversarial relationship between the malpractice attorney and the physician always looms in the background of medical decision making."

In other words, doctors must walk a tightrope between attending to their patient's welfare in a way they believe to be most beneficial while placating stressed-out family members as malpractice lawyers watch from the sidelines, ready to pounce. It is not what most doctors thought they were signing up for when they entered medical school. But it is the sad reality of American medicine.

Palliative-care physician David Weissman speaks candidly about the legal and psychological pressure placed on doctors who treat terminally ill patients, pressure that all too frequently compels them to extend a patient's life even if they know the patient is on the brink of natural death and that medical intervention will almost certainly lead to suffering. "Why should we expect clinicians to feel good about caring for the dying," Dr. Weissman asks rhetorically, "when they feel pressured, by the real or perceived threat of malpractice or institutional sanctions, to offer a medical procedure they know is not only useless, but downright harmful?"[2]

In his journal article, Dr. Weissman, who in addition to his medical duties teaches other doctors about EOL care issues, proposes a treatment model that if adopted might keep patients from falling into the death trap.

"I favor a hospital policy that links recognition of impending death to an institutional commitment to end of life care," he writes.[3] He suggests "the adoption of a formal family support/bereavement program that begins at the time death is anticipated."[4] His proposed treatment model would include "a mandatory visit by a palliative-care nurse/ team member to assess the adequacy of symptom control and [to initiate a] discussion of care setting options" with the patient or the patient's surrogate.[5]

It is worth noting that although Dr. Weissman proposed this model of care reform seventeen years ago, it still is not on anyone's reform radar. Wisdom and common sense, it seems, are no match for deeply entrenched institutional practices.

Sometimes neither the patient nor the patient's family nor the treating physician is prepared for the EOL decisions. That is when a doctor's training and instincts—and as you will see in this patient story, decency and compassion—come into play.

Ben, the cardiologist mentioned above, was the on-call cardiologist for a hospital ER one weekend when he received a 2 a.m. phone call summoning him to the hospital. When he arrived, he was asked to examine a critically ill patient who had been admitted to the ER with a suspected heart attack. The patient, he noted, was a "morbidly obese, 58-year-old man who was found on the floor next to his bed by his teenage daughter. She had started chest compressions and called 911. The rescue squad had incubated him in the field and brought him to the emergency room."

After examining the patient, recalls Ben, "it was clear that the mechanism of his collapse was not acute myocardial infarction (a heart attack) or an ongoing cardiac event," which was the ER doctor's mistaken diagnosis. "This patient's clinical evaluation, blood gas levels, and laboratory findings told him the grim news. He was fevered and unresponsive with grand mal brain seizure activity, accompanied by tonic-clonic muscular activity (stiffening and rhythmical twitching of the limbs)."

"The precise cause of his collapse," said Ben, "was never determined." However, "it did result in severe, irreversible, hypoxic brain injury, caused by a loss of oxygen to the brain, a condition that carries a very poor prognosis for survival.

After coming to this depressing conclusion, Ben now faced another quandary. How was he going to share the bad news with the patient's two teenage children while diplomatically explaining to them that the ER doctor, who had raised their hopes by suggesting that their father might be saved by a cardiac catheterization, had misdiagnosed their dad?

"I learned that the patient was a beloved teacher at a local high school," Ben told me.

> He was divorced and the sole caretaker for the seventeen-year-old daughter and fifteen-year-old son. They wanted to know why I wouldn't take their dad to the catheterization lab and save his life. Their expectations were unrealistic and created in part by the ER doctor's wanting to give them hope. No one wanted to tell these teenage children their father and sole caretaker was going to die. "I explained to them that a trip to the cath lab at this time could very

well make things worse, and the reality of their father's condition was grave."

"I spent well over an hour trying to console them and prepare them for the difficult decisions that lay ahead. These discussions were made even more challenging by the fact that the ER doctor had given them false hope that I was going to come to the rescue and provide some type of cure."

In recalling this experience, Ben reminded me of how vulnerable physicians are, even those like this highly regarded cardiologist who had been practicing for decades.

Dr. Leeat Granek coauthored a yearlong study on the psychological impact of losing a patient. The study included twenty oncologists treating cancer patients at three Canadian hospitals. According to Dr. Granek:

> We found that oncologists struggled to manage their feelings of grief with the detachment they felt was necessary to do their job. . . . More than half of our participants reported feelings of failure, self-doubt, sadness, and powerlessness as part of their grief experience, and a third talked about feelings of guilt, loss of sleep, and crying. Our study indicated that grief is considered shameful and unprofessional. Even though participants wrestled with feelings of grief, they hid them from others because showing emotion was considered a sign of weakness. In fact, many remarked that our interview was the first time they had been asked these questions or spoken about these emotions at all.[6]

"The impact of this unacknowledged grief," the researchers found, "was exactly what we don't want our doctors to experience: inattentiveness, impatience, emotional exhaustion and burnout."[7] "Even more distressing," asserted Granek, "half our participants reported that their discomfort with their grief over patient loss could affect their treatment decisions with subsequent patients—leading them, for instance, to provide more aggressive chemotherapy, to put a patient in a clinical trial, or recommend further surgery when palliative care might be a better option."[8]

Dr. Granek said she and her fellow researchers also found "a troubling relationship between doctors' discomfort with death and grief and how patients and their families are treated."[9] Their conclusion was that "to improve the quality of end of life care for patients and families, we need to improve the quality of life for physicians, by making space for them to grieve like everyone else."[10]

When examining the doctor's role at the end of life, one should keep in mind that a physician's training, desire to cure, and his or her unique values impact their treatment choices. For some professional healers, allowing a patient to die naturally may conflict with these factors that have molded them as physicians. For example, they may believe that human life is sacred, and this calls them to try and preserve that life at all costs. However, in *The Art of Dying Well*, journalist Katy Butler observes that doctors who insist on using all their technology trying to keep a patient alive are not necessarily engaging in an act of mercy. "Some doctors assume that everyone wants to extend life until there is no joy," she writes. "They are mistaken."[11]

Doctors often have a hard time letting people die. Discussing death with patients runs contrary to everything they were taught in medical school. The issue of extending a patient's life using high-tech treatments with little or no lasting benefit to the patient is addressed by surgeon and author Dr. Atul Gawande in his award-winning book *Being Mortal*. "Modern medicine," he states on the very first page, "is good at staving off death with aggressive interventions, and bad at knowing when to focus, instead, on improving the days the terminal patients have left."[12]

Dr. Gawande believes that the plight of physicians treating terminally ill patients is made even more onerous by the fact that so many of them, along with their families—and sometimes other doctors—are unwilling to face the bleak reality of their situation. As a result, ICUs across the country are filled with patients who will never leave the hospital alive.

"Recently, while seeing a patient in an intensive care unit at my hospital, I stopped to talk with the critical care physician on duty, someone I'd known since college. 'I am running a warehouse for the dying,' she said bleakly."[13] Out of ten patients in her unit, she told him, only two were likely to leave under their own power.

According to Gawande, this doctor's ICU patients included an eighty-year-old woman with irreversible congestive heart failure who was "drugged to oblivion and tubed in most natural orifices and a few artificial ones."[14] The physician also told Dr. Gawande about a seventy-year-old female patient with metastatic cancer who had chosen to forgo curative treatment but whose oncologist had "pushed her to change her mind, and she was put on a ventilator and antibiotics."[15] Perhaps the saddest case among this litany of the dying was that of a patient in her eighties with end-stage respiratory and kidney failure.

Dr. Gawande's physician friend told him that this patient's husband had "died after a long illness, with a feeding tube and a tracheotomy, and she had mentioned [to me] that she didn't want to die that way. But her children couldn't let her go, and asked [me] to proceed with the placement of various devices: a permanent tracheostomy, feeding tube and dialysis catheter."[16]

Because of these futile interventions, the dying patient "just lay there tethered to her pumps, drifting in and out of consciousness."[17] In his article, Dr. Gawande stressed that "almost all these patients had known, for some time, that they had a terminal condition. Yet they, along with their families and doctors, were unprepared for the final stage."[18]

Walking the thin line between life and death, doctors face multiple quandaries in treating dying patients and advising them and their loved ones about choices for EOL care. They need to be honest with their patients, but at the same time they need to be guarded in communicating to them the inevitability of their death.

One personal, and vivid, example of this tightrope involved an articulate daughter who shared with me she was furious with her grandmother's physician. Her grandmother was ninety years old and had congestive heart failure. The grandmother knew her time was limited and asked her physician how much time she had left. He responded honestly, saying it was probably not much more than six months. The granddaughter believed this honest response was entirely inappropriate because it would "take away hope and her grandmother's desire to live." When I indicated the physician's response seemed reasonable to me, she became indignant. However her perspective did heighten my own sensitivity to the role hope plays in EOL care.

Another patient story involving walking this thin line came from my wise and good friend Dr. David Leach.

I remember one of my first patients when I was a new medical staff member at Henry Ford Health System. I went to her room to deliver the news that she had inoperable lung cancer. She asked how long she had. I told her that no one could answer that, that she might even die of something else, but that lung cancer would be with her when she died. She replied, "Dr. Leach you are a nice guy but you are not very helpful. I have two books here, a collection of short stories and a two-volume edition of *War and Peace*. Which should I start reading?" We laughed and I saw her courage and dignity, she saw that I saw, and it comforted both of us. End-of-life care should allot time for acknowledging the person's uniqueness, it should help them make sense of their lives. It's good for the patient and the caregiver.

"To discuss dying with a patient is sad work," notes Ann Neumann. "Doctors have to admit their inability to cure whatever disease is ending a patient's life."[19] Moreover, Ms. Neumann says patients and families don't want to hear a pessimistic diagnosis. Patients and families resist the truth, and they don't make it easy for doctors to be candid.

Dr. Ezekiel Emanuel asserts that "talking about end of life is the hardest thing a doctor does. It is emotionally charged, it is physically draining, it takes time, and we need to recognize that increasingly these conversations require a lot of skill. These are not physical skills, manual skills or dexterity, but it is about something just as important. It's about emotional understanding of patients and it ought to be compensated the way we compensate for other skills and talents."[20]

Regrettably, the healthcare payment system in this country does not compensate physicians adequately for having this conversation with patients. Even if a higher-paid billing code were created for such conversations, these conversations are unlikely to ever be the same and fit neatly into a code. In 2020 the average visit with a primary care doctor in the United States lasted for about fourteen minutes. That is not enough time to have meaningful conversation about EOL care—or for that matter, about anything at all.

There is a cultural reason that training of physicians on EOL counseling is not a priority for U.S. medical schools. New technology, research, and treatments for curing patients are the focus of medical school curricula because these are the American healthcare system's priorities.

The reality is that physicians do not have a cure for chronic illnesses and the inevitable aging process. The healthcare system is unprepared to provide social support for the frail elderly that are growing exponentially in this country. What these patients need is social support and education about what to expect while aging. What we give them is high-tech healthcare. This situation is largely due to our society's economic incentives and ethical priorities. Individuals come to their physicians with social support problems, and the primary tool kit available to the physician is high-tech treatment.

Medical school deans, healthcare leaders, and our government should recognize the urgency of changing our approach to responding to one of the most formidable challenges that we face: comforting and guiding patients in their final days.

In the end, however, some of my doctor friends have told me, even the best-trained or most experienced physician can find themselves overwhelmed at times by the responsibility of caring for a dying patient. Their predicament was eloquently captured by Dr. Dan Sulmasy, author and professor of biomedical ethics at Georgetown University, reflecting on the difficulty of supporting patients as they approach death. "It should be a challenge to decide when it is time to forgo further life-sustaining treatments," he writes.[21]

> To make such a decision means that a genuine someone (a mother, or a sister or a grandfather, or some other child of God) will die, and that is always bad, always a loss, even when the decision is right and true and just. Such judgements must take into account the particulars of the individual patient and those who love her, the nature of the disease, the way it has affected this patient, and a host of other circumstances.[22]

Summing up the physician's plight in advising a dying patient about when to let go, Sulmasy observes that "helping a patient to arrive at such a decision can be a powerful experience that reverberates with all the dignity of the human."[23] I believe he speaks for all doctors when he admits that regardless of the individual circumstances, guiding a patient along the final step "is never easy."

Nurse and author Sallie Tisdale in *Advice for Future Corpses* observes that "when a physician allows a patient to die naturally, they are doing the right thing. When we take a terminally ill patient off life support," she writes, "we are not pulling the plug, we are freeing the patient to die. We are releasing them from excessive technology and invasive treatments. When we allow death to happen, we are not killing people, we are caring for them. We are loving them."[24]

We need to allow physicians time to care for their patients. We also need to rebalance the physician relationship and create a more explicit duty for physicians to discuss death with their patients.

7

PATIENT AUTONOMY

A Double-Edged Sword

> Every human being of adult years and sound mind has the
> right to determine what shall be done with his own body.
>
> —New York Appeals Court Justice Benjamin Cardozo
> in *Schloendorff v. Society of New York Hospital*, 1914

In this book's second chapter you learned about the many reasons that curative care has become the default treatment option for EOL care in America. You may recall that one of those reasons was the insistence by patients or their family members that they receive every available medical intervention to prolong their life. In the United States, patients have the legal right, under a medical ethics principle known as "patient autonomy," to demand such treatment regardless of the cost even if the intervention they seek has a nominal chance of restoring them to health. Under this treatment paradigm, the patient, rather than his or her physician, has become the final arbiter of the medical care he or she will receive.

This right of patient autonomy, one of the bedrock principles of medical ethics, has progressively evolved over the last one hundred years. Before this time, physicians dominated care decisions for patients. This power shift, which was needed, has unfortunately become a double-edged sword and particularly in EOL care. Gravely ill patients suffer more than they need to, and billions of dollars are wasted every year on expensive and often futile medical interventions. How, one might reasonably ask, did this radical reversal of roles between the doctor and the patient come about?

"Informed consent" evolved from patient autonomy. This legal concept emerged in the 1940s and 1950s in response to public outrage over research projects conducted by U.S. medical professionals who were testing unproven treatments on patients without their consent. The researchers rationalized their surreptitious medical experiments by asserting that their studies were essential to advancing medicine.[1] They said the potential dangers to which their human guinea pigs unwittingly were being exposed were necessary to make those advances. That rationale, conceived during an era in which physicians were vested with nearly limitless authority and deemed by society as virtually above reproach, was wrong. Doctors no longer enjoy an untouchable status in our society, and using patients as research subjects without the patient's knowledge or consent is now prohibited.

HOW DO PATIENT AUTONOMY AND INFORMED CONSENT WORK?

Essentially, patient autonomy means being in control of your own medical decisions without outside influence. Your physician is obliged to explain your treatment options along with their associated clinical risks and potential benefits. He or she then must obtain your informed consent to administer the treatment you have chosen. The concept is relatively simple and straightforward. Applying it to real-world circumstances, however, can be challenging. Choices about medical care are complex and often difficult to understand. Some healthcare providers have attempted to address this issue by turning the decision-making process into an educational experience.

This approach worked well in the health crisis I faced a few years ago, which was successfully addressed with open-heart surgery. Following my diagnosis, I was shown a thirty-minute educational video explaining the risks and benefits of the procedure as well as details of the surgery and recovery process. After viewing the video, I had some time to reflect on what I'd learned before sitting down to discuss my questions and concerns with the cardiac team that would later perform the procedure. The educational video, followed up by my meeting with the surgical team, not only allowed me to give my informed consent without any qualms but also increased my confidence in my caregivers and allowed me to go into surgery with a positive mindset.

To be honest, however, my decision to undergo this high-risk medical procedure involved a lot more than educating myself about its risks and meeting the medical professionals who would carry it out. Like anyone else faced with such a dilemma, I was scared. I had a lot to think about. On the upside, replacing the clogged arteries could improve the quality of my life. But I also had to contemplate the potential downsides of the surgery. For instance, I had to confront the possibility that I could become part of the 2 percent of heart bypass patients who die on the operating table each year. Or I could suffer a stroke, causing brain damage that would leave me in a severely compromised physical state for the balance of my days. To me, losing my faculties, by which I mean the ability to think clearly, carry out such routine daily tasks as bathing, eating, or going to the toilet under my own power—and most importantly, connecting meaningfully with those I hold dear—would be far worse than dying.

Put simply, when you are facing a medical crisis you might not survive, patient autonomy becomes a lot more than an abstract term describing a decision-making process. You will be asked to make decisions that could determine not only whether you will live or die but the quality of your life should you have the opportunity to extend it. If you are gravely ill, you may be forced to ask yourself, Am I willing to suffer the physical pain or mental confusion brought on by heroic medical interventions that could buy me a little more time? Am I ready to surrender to the natural process of dying? Am I willing to confront my fear and uncertainty about death? These are some of the questions you will be called upon to answer during a medical crisis such as the one I faced in 2017. Because of patient autonomy, for better or worse, you will have the final word on the nature, and limits, of the medical care you will receive. Are you prepared to take on this responsibility? Hopefully what you learn in the pages of this book will help you more confidently and effectively use your patient power.

PATIENT EMPOWERMENT

Unfortunately, my positive experience with surgery was not necessarily typical—particularly for EOL situations. Many patients and families do not understand the implications of the care they will receive. In addition, they may be poorly informed about other options of care available to them such as hospice and palliative care. Or they may not *want* to exercise their patient autonomy. I remember, for example, people in my parents' generation, including my parents themselves, wanting little to do with this new legal right. They preferred having their doctors tell them what to do. It was what their parents had done, and it felt right and comfortable to them to do the same.

The problem is that even when dealing with patients who are willing to take an active role in their medical treatment, doctors sometimes do a poor job of providing them with a holistic understanding of their treatment options and risks. To be fair, educating patients who are elderly or gravely ill can be difficult under the best of circumstances. And as you might imagine, it becomes a lot more challenging in the middle of a health crisis. When a person's life is at stake, his or her interest in asserting patient autonomy or exercising the right to refuse a proposed medical procedure understandably diminishes. At this point, most patients are willing to accept any treatment they believe may save their life.

DWINDLING CHOICES

At the end of life we tend to have fewer effective healthcare treatment options. Quite often the patient finds himself looking at the pros and cons of a single recommended procedure from a medical specialist's perspective. This rarely benefits the patient. For example, the surgery the specialist proposes may cure gangrene or open a blocked artery, but if the patient is dying anyway, the best outcome one could expect would be a bit more time. On the other hand, the cure may also turn the patient's existence into a living hell. Remember the example given in chapter 2 of the retired school nurse whose infected leg was amputated but who died after much suffering only a few days later. The nephew of the patient, who held healthcare power of attorney (HCPA), approved the amputation surgery. But vicariously exercising his aunt's patient autonomy while acting as her medical surrogate turned out to be a curse for her rather than a blessing. At the end of the day, what matters is how a patient or her surrogate uses their autonomy, a decision-making power that can best be described as a double-edged sword.

RACIAL DISPARITY AND ITS IMPACT ON PATIENT AUTONOMY CONVERSATIONS

It is well documented that African Americans facing a terminal illness are less likely than whites to choose hospice care.[2] The reasons are certainly understandable and go back to the well-known Tuskegee study. This study allowed African American men to die so clinicians could study the progression of a curable disease. These men were intentionally allowed to die in the name of medical research.

More recently, research has documented poorer healthcare outcomes for minorities.[3] One of the more flagrant examples is that the fetal mortality rate for African Americans is double the national average.[4] The consequences of these outcomes has resulted in understandable distrust and suspicion of healthcare in the African American community.

It does not take much imagination to envision how these patients will react to a white male physician suggesting to them that not pursuing further medical treatment is in their best interest. Offering patients the alternative to die naturally with hospice may come across as more like denying African Americans needed healthcare.

Unfortunately, few clinicians have the skill set or time required to discuss these issues with the sensitivity they deserve. The ability to openly discuss death with a patient is never easy. Add the complexity of cultural nuances to the conversation and it becomes even more delicate. Clinicians are not adequately prepared to appreciate that people from different cultures have diverse and varying reactions to understanding their treatment options. Enhanced sensitivity is needed in handling these conversations and is particularly significant for EOL discussions. Patients deserve cultural sensitivity. Without it, most patients will not have the opportunity to really learn about their options and then give their informed consent. The resulting communication breakdowns hurt these patients and hamper their ability to knowledgeably exercise their autonomy.

The issue of racial disparity in healthcare goes well beyond the purview of this book. The point being made is that racial disparity surfaces in EOL care because these patients don't trust the health system. Therefore these patients miss out on the benefits of selecting hospice and a natural death because their patient autonomy is exercised without proper informed consent.

THE PROS AND CONS OF PATIENT AUTONOMY

In theory patient autonomy is a humane, just, even enlightened concept. However as noted by Jesuit ethicist Father John J. Paris, some of its flaws are substantial. Father Paris suggests that empowering patients to effectively dictate their treatment has substantially increased healthcare spending.[5] Moreover, it has transformed the traditional doctor-patient relationship from a joint venture of trust and dependency into a unilateral, patient-directed treatment model.

"The morphing of the right of the competent patient to decline an unwanted medical intervention into the right to be provided whatever medical intervention [he or she desires] indifferent to efficacy or cost," argues Father Paris, "results in . . . the chaos of present-day healthcare delivery in the United States."[6] Moreover, says the Jesuit ethicist, "when the rightness or wrongness of a decision is reduced to an individual [patient's] choice, the result is autonomy gone amok."[7] Such an approach, he asserts, "gives no consideration to the impact individual choices have on family and friends [of the patient], the medical profession, or society."[8]

By "society" Father Paris seems to be referring to our obligation as taxpayers to fund the constantly expanding costs of our national healthcare system. If every dying patient in an American hospital demanded that every possible means be used to keep him or her alive as long as possible, the financial consequences would be staggering, and eventually it would bankrupt the healthcare system.

Thankfully bankruptcy has not happened—yet. But the potential for it happening underlines the need to approach patient autonomy in a more balanced and holistic manner so that the patient, family members, caregivers, and the American taxpayer all will benefit. Admittedly in today's healthcare culture, which incentivizes consumption and focuses on cures, introducing this more holistic model for patient autonomy by balancing multiple interests will be challenging. One of the biggest hurdles will be changing society's expectations of doctors. Physicians are taught that patient autonomy should always be paramount. They defer to the patient's wishes or the patient's family's wishes even if they believe the requested treatment will do more harm than good. They do this in part because of the ever-present danger of being sued by the patient's family for not doing enough to save their loved one. But they also want to respect their patient's wishes, which in today's patient-centric medical culture are virtually sacrosanct. The problem with this treatment approach is that it too often leads to needless suffering.

When government officials enter the fray, the inherent flaws in the patient autonomy model become more glaring. For instance, during the administration of President Jimmy Carter, well-meaning healthcare bureaucrats decided that we should deinstitutionalize mental patients and, to the extent possible, empty out the nation's psychiatric hospitals and wards. Anyone who was paying attention—either back then or now—can see that the state, local, and federal healthcare officials who were supposed to provide outpatient counseling and meds to these liberated patients have almost totally failed. These mentally disturbed individuals, many of whom are schizophrenic, addicted to drugs or alcohol, military veterans suffering from post-traumatic stress disorder, or all the above, now make up most of our country's burgeoning homeless population. On the other hand, they have unlimited autonomy.

ALFIE'S STORY

The difficulty of striking an acceptable balance among the three principal parties to patient autonomy—the patient, the patient's family, and the healthcare provider—is poignantly illustrated by the story of Alfie Evans, a toddler who died in an English hospital in April 2018 after being removed from a ventilator against his parents' wishes.

His sad story began in December 2016 when Alfie, then just seven months old, was admitted to the Alder Hey Children's Hospital in

Liverpool, England, after experiencing a series of unexplained seizures. Staff physicians discovered he was suffering from a rare brain disorder characterized by progressive neurological degeneration. He was placed on a ventilator to assist his breathing and he received nutrition through a feeding tube.

Over the next year, his condition gradually worsened. According to hospital physicians, scans of Alfie's brain showed that this diminutive patient had sustained "catastrophic degradation of his brain tissue" due to his malady, known as GABA-transaminase deficiency.[9] The doctors advised Alfie's parents, Tom Evans and Kate James, that due to the brain damage their son had sustained, any further medical treatment would be futile. They said that continuing to keep Alfie alive through artificial means would be "unkind and inhumane." For this reason, they told the child's grieving parents they were going to take Alfie off life support.

The parents, who against all odds, still held out hope for their son's miraculous recovery, objected to the move. They then embarked on an epic legal battle to keep their son on life support, going all the way to the Supreme Court of the United Kingdom. Ultimately, they lost their legal battle after a judge ruled that "the hospital must be free to do what has been determined [by its staff physicians] to be in Alfie's best interests."

The ruling infuriated Tom Evans, who insisted, "[Alfie] isn't suffering, he isn't in pain, he isn't diagnosed [as clinically brain dead]." Evans added, bitterly, "It's a straight-up execution."

The Evans family appealed to the pope, who responded very sympathetically by offering care for Alfie at Bambino Gesù Hospital in Rome free of charge. Unfortunately Alfie's medical team and the courts in England were unwilling to release Alfie to pursue this alternative care option. They believed it was not in Alfie's best interest. Given Alfie's age and the parent's firmly held belief, it is hard to understand why the Evans family were denied the right to pursue this option.

Good versus Evil

The media, of course, recognized a compelling human drama when they saw one. Journalists on both sides of the Atlantic framed the story as a battle between the forces of good (Alfie and his parents) and evil (the English courts and hospital physicians and leaders). Shortly before

Alfie died on April 25, 2018, a few days after being removed from life support, Dr. Betsy McCaughey published a story in the *New York Post* in which she bluntly stated, "The hospital is dooming [Alfie] to die."[10] She then cited the cases of two other English children who had expired after being removed from life support against their parents' wishes. Indeed, she all but accused the hospital physicians of murdering these youngsters when she stated, "Alfie isn't the first child sentenced to die by a British hospital."[11]

Using such inflammatory language to stir up public outrage makes for dramatic headlines, but in the end, accusing doctors, who are acting in what they believe is in their patient's best interest, of murdering someone benefits no one. The fact is that healthcare providers are sometimes called upon to decide how much additional medical treatment should be provided to an unresponsive patient with little realistic hope of physical recovery. In little Alfie's case, I'm sure that taking him off life support was an agonizing decision for his doctors to make. They believed they were ethically obliged to spare this youngster from experiencing protracted physical discomfort and pain that fulfilled no healing purpose. Despite amazing advances in medical knowledge and technology, the sad fact is doctors cannot save everyone—no matter how much they might wish otherwise.

Around two weeks before Alfie Evans passed away, a group of impassioned supporters, dubbed "Alfie's Army" by the British press, gathered near the entrance to the Alder Hey Children's Hospital to protest the healthcare facility's decision to take Alfie off of life support. Convinced that both the ailing child and his parents were being treated unjustly, even cruelly, by the English medical establishment, they accused hospital staff members who emerged from the building of trying to kill the little boy. However, they backed off when local law enforcement officials warned them that the next person who made a verbal threat against a hospital employee would be arrested and criminally prosecuted.

As a former member of the professional healthcare community, my heart goes out to the doctors, nurses, and hospital administrators who were caught in the crossfire of an unwinnable fight. These caregivers and hospital officials risked a great deal by making the decision to take Alfie off the ventilator and feeding tube. They were doing what they believed was right.

My heart equally goes out to the Evans family who worked so hard to find Alfie an alternative care option in Rome and were denied their right to pursue this alternative.

THE FIGHT OVER PATIENT AUTONOMY CONTINUES

Similar legal battles over who has the right to decide when a patient can be removed from life support also have been fought in American courtrooms—most famously in the cases of Karen Ann Quinlan (1976), Nancy Cruzan (1990), and Terri Schiavo (2005). All three young women sustained irreversible brain damage and were being kept alive by means of a feeding tube or ventilator. In all three cases, patient autonomy was the central issue.

The Cruzan case was similar to Alfie's story. The significant difference was that the courts prevented the family from taking their daughter *off* life support. In a precedent-setting 1990 ruling in *Cruzan v. Director, Missouri Department of Health*, the U.S. Supreme Court upheld the State of Missouri's claim that it had both the right and the responsibility to decide what was in a comatose patient's best interest.[12] (See chapter 9 for a more detailed discussion of this controversial case.) In the state's eyes, that meant keeping Missouri resident Nancy Cruzan, who had sustained irreversible brain injury in a car crash, alive indefinitely through artificial means. Cruzan's parents eventually convinced a trial judge to let them take her off life support, which they then did, allowing her to die peacefully soon thereafter.

The Cruzan case was covered intensively by the media, sparking a national debate over the legal rights of a patient who cannot make critical medical decisions for him- or herself. That debate in turn led to the passage of the 1990 Patient Self-Determination Act, a federal law enacted in support of patient autonomy. Under this law, which took effect December 1, 1991, all healthcare facilities receiving Medicare or Medicaid insurance payments are required to inform their newly admitted patients in writing about their right to choose the medical treatments they will receive at the end of life and about the nature of those treatments. These medical institutions are also required to inform patients of their right to create a living will or AHD spelling out their

EOL treatment preferences. Because one of the main purposes of the law is to prevent "cruel overtreatment for profit of elderly [Medicare and Medicaid patients]," those instructions should include the medical measures these highly vulnerable patients do *not* wish to be undertaken to extend their lives.

According to an article published in October 1993, a study showed that while applying this law in a hospital setting "increased patient awareness of living wills, [it] failed to increase the number of patients who act on this awareness."[13] In other words, even when elderly or gravely ill patients are informed of their patient autonomy rights, many prefer not to take any action. Who can blame them? As discussed earlier in this book, no one likes to think about their own susceptibility to illness, suffering, or death until or unless they absolutely must. All of the laws in the world, including the Patient Self-Determination Act, cannot change this fundamental tenet of human nature.

Admittedly the bitterly contested legal battles discussed in this chapter are unusual and atypical of EOL scenarios played out every day in hospitals and nursing homes across England and the United States. However, they contain valuable lessons. First, they demonstrate that not much good happens when courts get involved in arbitrating life-and-death medical decisions. Asking judicial officials who are unschooled in medical complexities to balance conflicting views on EOL care is never a good idea. The Alfie Evans and Nancy Cruzan cases also show how the media can sensationalize sensitive medical dilemmas, making it even more difficult for all parties involved in such disputes to make reasoned choices.

COVID-19 AND IVERMECTIN

Ivermectin is an antiparasitic treatment commonly used for livestock and humans infected by parasitic worms. In mid-2021, this medication gained traction as a treatment for the COVID-19 delta variant outbreak. This traction was not based on proven scientific research but instead on endorsements by politicians and public personalities. This potential conflict evolved into a battle over patient autonomy.

A fifty-one-year-old patient named Jeffery Smith came down with COVID-19 in July 2021 and was hospitalized at a University of Cincinnati hospital. His wife of twenty-four years, Julie Smith, asked on August 20 for an emergency court order to allow her husband to be treated with ivermectin by a physician not associated with the hospital.

Initially Judge Gregory Howard authorized Dr. Fred Wagshul to treat Jeffrey Smith with 30 milligrams of ivermectin daily for three weeks. Mr. Smith had been sedated, intubated, and on a ventilator for three weeks. The hospital appealed to a higher court for a reversal of the order. The physicians did not believe this course of treatment was in their patient's best interest.

The appellate court reversed the order and ruled that the hospital's physicians could not be compelled to administer ivermectin. Specifically, the opinion stated,

> Everyone involved wants Jeffrey Smith to get better. Simply stated, there are no bad actors in this case. [Judge Michael Oster Jr. said it is] impossible not to feel sympathetic [for this family but he must rule against their request]. . . . The FDA, CDC, AMA, AphAA and the doctors at this hospital do not believe ivermectin should be used to treat COVID–19. . . . Oster also said the doctor who testified about Jeffrey Smith's condition could only say "he seemed to be getting better." . . . Oster also said that Jeffery Smith could be moved to another hospital where the drug could be administered.[14]

Approximately one month after these court decisions, the patient died. Nevertheless, conflicts over patient autonomy, such as the story above, illustrate the tension and angst created when third parties attempt to exercise this most personal of rights.

These cases should be motivation for all of us to educate ourselves about our EOL care options when our minds are clear and we are not in pain, frightened, unconscious, or fighting to stay alive and to spell out our preferences in an AHD. This is the ultimate expression of patient autonomy.

8

WHO'S AFRAID OF
THE BIG, BAD GR?

I sleep with life and death in the same bed.

—Bob Dylan

In countless cartoons and works of art, the grim reaper (GR) is depicted as a scary-looking skeleton typically wearing a black cape and hood. He carries a scythe and is not the kind of individual you'd want to hang around with—especially at harvest time. Sooner or later, however, we're all going to have to confront the GR. Ideally, we will be able to do this in a way that empowers us and not him. We can put the odds squarely on our side by preparing ourselves for the inevitable.

We can manage our stage exit well by making clear, educated choices early. Or more typically, we'll avoid planning for or even thinking about our final days and let our fear of death overwhelm us. This would not make us cowards. Nor would it make us foolish. It would make us human.

In her groundbreaking 1969 book *On Death and Dying*, Swiss-American psychiatrist Elisabeth Kübler-Ross asserts that humans instinctively avoid death. It is a fate we universally refuse to face. Kübler-Ross notes that many of the terminally ill hospital patients she interviewed in compiling her psychological study were in denial; that is, they either could not or would not accept the grim reality of their predicament.[1] She codified this psychological response as the first of five consecutive stages of grief experienced by the dying. The four succeeding stages she identified were anger (at the injustice of their fate); bargaining (for more time or a chance to complete essential life goals); depression (at realizing they could not escape death); and finally, acceptance, a resignation to the inevitable that lightens the patient's psychological burden and in some cases allows the patient to experience an extraordinary sense of peace and liberation. In a memorable passage from the book, Kübler-Ross poignantly describes her own experience witnessing the death of such a patient.

> Those who have the strength and the love to sit with a dying patient in the silence that goes beyond words will know that this moment is neither frightening nor painful but a peaceful cessation of the body's functioning. Watching the peaceful death of a human being reminds us of a falling star, one of a million lights in a vast sky that flares up for a brief moment.[2]

In the more than half century that has passed since her book's publication, critics have challenged Kübler-Ross's "arbitrary," perhaps even unfounded, theory of discrete psychological stages, but her work is arguably the first in-depth analysis, from a physician's perspective, of death's emotional implications. She brought this taboo topic into the open and began a lively dialogue on death and dying that continues to this day.

CIVILIZATION AND THE FEAR OF DEATH

According to Ernst Becker, an American cultural anthropologist, our lives are an unconscious response to our fear of death. In his Pulitzer Prize–winning book *The Denial of Death*, published just four years after *On Dying and Death*, Becker states what few honest people, including Elizabeth Kübler-Ross, would contest; namely, that "the idea of death, the fear of it, haunts the human animal like nothing else."[3] But Becker also credits this psychological bogeyman with being the main creative force behind civilization. The terror sparked by the realization of our mortality, he says, "is a mainspring of human activity—activity designed largely to avoid the fatality of death, to overcome it by denying it in some way."[4]

In his book, Becker discusses the psychological strategies we use to construct denial mechanisms, strategies he calls "immortality projects."[5] According to Becker, these allow us to function in the world as if we will not die. This very productive act of self-delusion is possible, says Becker, because greater society "creates a hero system that allows us to believe that we transcend death by participating in something of lasting worth. We achieve ersatz immortality by sacrificing ourselves to conquer an empire, to build a temple, to write a book, to establish a family, to accumulate a fortune, to further progress and prosperity."[6]

TERROR MANAGEMENT

Three American social psychologists—Sheldon Solomon, Jeff Greenberg, and Tom Pyszczynski—were so taken by Becker's insights regarding our unconscious response to the fear of death they spent the next quarter of a century investigating this phenomenon. Their voluminous research, culminating in the publication of *The Worm at the Core* in 2015, explored what they call "terror management," a psychological concept that builds on Becker's intellectual foundations. "Our overarching goals," they said, "are to reveal [the] many ways [in which] the knowledge that we are mortal underlies both the noblest and the most unsavory of human pursuits and to consider how these insights can lead to personal growth and social progress."[7]

These researchers were particularly interested in the roles that ritual, art, myth, and religion play in helping us overcome our fear of death by giving us hope for immortality. Concerning religion's role in subduing our worries, they observed,

> Throughout the ages, the vast majority of people . . . have been led by their religions to believe that their existence continues in some form beyond physical death. Some of us believe that our souls fly up to heaven. . . . Others "know" that at the moment of death, our souls migrate into a new, reincarnated form. Still others are convinced that our souls pass to another, unknown plane of existence. In all these cases, we believe that we are . . . literally immortals.[8]

In their twenty-five-year investigation, the trio of social psychologists worked on over five hundred studies to demonstrate "the many ways that cultural worldviews protect us from the terror that the knowledge of the inevitability of death might otherwise arouse."[9] They concluded that our psychological well-being depends on our belief that we are valuable contributors to a meaningful world—a view reinforced by the rest of society, who are busy carrying out their own immortality projects. This belief, the authors say, "fortified" our ancestors against the fear of death and simultaneously drove the engine of human progress.

Art, myth, rituals, and religions provided a sense of protection and immortality to our ancestors. As such, our ancestors were psychologically fortified and could take full advantage of their sophisticated mental abilities. They deployed them to develop the belief systems, technology, and science that ultimately propelled us into the modern world.

THE DOWNSIDE OF FEAR

If our evolving civilization is the astonishing by-product of our existential fear, what, one might ask, is the downside of this mindset? Frankly, there are far too many such negatives to discuss in a single chapter. But if asked to name the single most destructive aspect of the impact of this fear, I would point to the needless suffering caused by the largely futile medical interventions made at the end of life. Often these interventions are due to a patient's, or the patient's family's, perfectly understandable but sometimes tragically misguided quest to postpone death. At best, they briefly extend the dying patient's stay in the world, but at what cost?

This issue is thoroughly investigated by sisters Jeanne and Eileen Fitzpatrick in *A Better Way of Dying*. They assert that "our society's fear of death is causing untold suffering for the dying and their families."[10] To address this issue, they came up with an approach to EOL medical care they call the "compassion protocol," which they describe as a "tool to heal the impasse between [the physician's Hippocratic Oath of] Do No Harm and Please let me die."[11]

In their book, the Fitzpatrick sisters explain that their protocol "guides the dying and their family members through a simple set of steps to obtain a Natural Death."[12] The steps may be simple, but they are not necessarily easy. To complete the first step, for example, the patient must decide they are "ready to die."

The remaining steps for those seeking a natural death are somewhat less imposing. For example, the individual needs to clarify that they do not want to be taken to the hospital for curative treatment of simple illnesses. They also need to declare their right to refuse antibiotics, hydration, and nutrition and to stop taking medications.

Also included in the book as appendix A is a five-page Compassion Protocol Contract, which the patient—or anyone reading the book— can copy, fill out, sign, and provide copies of to prospective caretakers. On the form, those seeking a natural rather than a mechanized death must specify, for example, whether they wish to be resuscitated if they stop breathing. They also are asked to answer a series of questions about their state of mind such as "Am I ready to let death happen?"[13] These questions are designed to determine if the patient is opting for death because of clear, rational thinking or as a result of depression. The form reflects the wisdom and humanity of the authors, who say they created the compassion protocol because they had seen too many people suffer needlessly at the end of their life. Their goal in publishing the protocol and the book was to help dying patients—or people planning for their eventual EOL care—overcome their fear of death by informing them about their care choices and offering them a chance to take control of their final journey.

FAITH CAN PLAY A ROLE

Others investigating people's attitudes toward death have found that a strong faith in God is associated with both emotional well-being and low death anxiety. The truth of this finding was driven home to me personally when I saw how my father, Francis Gough Connelly, a man of deep religious faith, responded to a series of devastating medical setbacks starting four years after he retired.

My father and I were very close. He was kind, thoughtful, and intuitive. I believe his kindness came from his belief that we are all equal in God's eyes. He spoke simply and straightforwardly. He had no pretense. He had exceptional people skills and was well liked by those who worked with him. However he did have his weaknesses as a father and husband. For example, he was reluctant to engage in the everyday demands of family life, particularly financial obligations. Being close to him meant I chose to overlook his flaws.

For fifteen years my father served as the county administrator of Monroe County, Wisconsin, working out of Sparta, the county seat. He then took a job in the personnel department of St. Mary's Hospital in Milwaukee. At age sixty-seven, after twenty-five years at St. Mary's, he retired from his post as assistant administrator of the hospital. However in an unusual post-retirement arrangement, he was given a small office to use. In return for a modest stipend, he acted as the hospital's unofficial ambassador, representing St. Mary's at community meetings and other events including funerals for staff physicians and other hospital employees. Anyone who worked for St. Mary's was considered a member of this traditional Catholic medical institution's family.

On February 10, 1980, my dad suffered a stroke. He was in his office at the hospital. He called a junior hospital administrator to whom he had become close and asked him if he could drive him home. Fortunately, seeing my dad's condition, the young man ignored his request and took him immediately to the ER.

At the time my dad was seventy-one years old. That day in the ER would mark the first time he had ever been treated or even examined by a doctor. Ironically, this longtime hospital employee was pretty much a Christian Scientist when it came to seeking medical care. He believed that in most cases our bodies naturally heal themselves. Regrettably this was not one of those cases. The skilled physicians at St. Mary's got him through his medical crisis. However, he had suffered brain damage from the stroke. After spending four months in a rehab facility, he was sent home to live with my mother. He was able to walk with a cane but spoke with a slur.

For the next four years, my father enjoyed a limited but nonetheless fulfilling life. He attended my graduation from law school. This was a big day for both of us. My dad had always wanted me to be a lawyer. He was a fan of Clarence Darrow, the legendary trial lawyer who saved the infamous Chicago child killers Leopold and Loeb from hanging and who defended Tennessee school teacher John Scopes, accused of teaching his students Darwin's theory of evolution (which went against the state's Bible-based creationist curriculum). Clearly, I had a lot to live up to if Clarence Darrow was to be my role model. The law degree, obtained at my dad's insistence, became a great asset when combined with a focus on healthcare management.

At the age of seventy-four, my father's overall health began to decline. He developed cataracts. He decided to have cataract surgery. Although it is a routine procedure, due to his previous stroke the risk for complications were real. Still he wanted the procedure done. Reading newspapers was one of his last remaining pleasures, and this required good eyesight. Unfortunately he suffered another stroke shortly after the surgery and was readmitted to the hospital. His doctor told him he would be bed-bound for the rest of his days. My mother was too fragile to care for him at their home, so we had to consider placing him in a nursing home.

I will never forget touring several such facilities in Milwaukee with my brother James. After those demoralizing visits, we both knew a nursing home was not a viable option. Our restless, independent father would never accept being physically helpless and dependent on others for his comfort and survival. Nor would he want to become a burden on anyone.

I discussed the situation with my dad. I offered to have him come live with my family in Chicago. He declined.

"That would not be good for your family," he responded.

I knew in my heart he was right. But other than moving in with me or another of his adult children, what other choice did my father have? As if reading my thoughts, he told me he was going to die in his hospital where he had worked for a quarter of a century.

There was no hospice option in those days at St. Mary's. Though my dad never revealed this to me, I believe he'd had a conversation with his physician, a friend and an old-school family practitioner, when he concluded he was close to the end. He stayed in the hospital for over three weeks. This violated Medicare rules, but the hospital officials made an exception for my father, who was a revered and beloved figure at St. Mary's. He basically used the hospital as a hospice. He had no more tests or therapy done. He took no medicines. He stopped eating and drinking even though he was offered sustenance every day. Essentially, he followed all the precepts of the compassion protocol—twenty-six years before they were formalized by the Fitzpatrick sisters in *A Better Way of Dying*.

His siblings visited—all six of them. They, along with my mother, brother, sister, and I, had some wonderful bedside conversations with my dad. I drafted a will for him using the legal knowledge and skills he had urged me to acquire.

When his turn came with the GR, Francis Connelly did so with dignity and courage. He had decided how he was going to meet his Maker. He never wavered from his plan. His attitude toward dying, I believe, reflected his stoic nature and his Irish Catholic upbringing. Stoicism is a centuries-old philosophy, a set of beliefs by which you accept—quietly and without complaint—what life gives you (incidentally, this attitude greatly influenced my upbringing, and indeed forged my character). A stoic interpretation of life would be as follows: God decides when you will die. He prepares a place for you in the after-life, but it is up to you to decide how you will live . . . and how you will face the end of your days.

On August 25, 1985, my father died, naturally and on his own terms, in a setting that had become like a second home to him. St. Mary's later named a meeting room in his honor. In retrospect I suspect there were moments, when death was near, that fear crept into my father's heart. But he was able to call upon his courage and his faith to overcome it.

One of my fondest memories growing up was our family reunion in Darlington, Wisconsin. This was the farming town where my father and mother grew up. We would go to my dad's home, where his parents hosted the reunion for their seven children and twenty-two grandchildren. We would dig to China, play sports, visit farms, go horseback riding at our cousin's farm, and sing songs together. At the end of a full day, we would all gather on the first floor of the house to pray the rosary led by Sr. Raymond Connelly, my dad's oldest sister. Perhaps the rosary was a source of strength for my father as he faced the last stage of life.

Let me close this chapter with a reflection from my good friend Dr. David Leach:

> I have found the Sorrowful Mysteries of the Rosary helpful in considering the end of life. Each mystery highlights a particular aspect of dying that must be dealt with by both the patient and the caregiver. The First Mystery is The Agony (anxiety/apprehension), The Second Mystery is The Scourging (pain), The Third Mystery is the Crowning of the Thornes (humiliation), The Fourth Mystery is

The Carrying of the Cross (endurance) and the Fifth Mystery is the Crucifixion (resignation).[14]

This remarkable reflection of faith is amazingly similar to Dr. Kübler-Ross's research on the five stages of dying and perhaps offers all of us thoughts worthy of reflection.

9

DISAPPEARING

A human being would certainly not grow to be seventy
or eighty years old if this longevity had no meaning for
the species to which he belongs. The afternoon of human
life must also have a significance of its own and cannot be
merely a pitiful appendage to life's morning.

—Carl Jung

When you reach a certain age in America, chances are you will acquire at least one superpower: invisibility. Our cultural approach
to age and infirmity is to isolate the sick and elderly in hospitals, nursing
homes, rehabilitation facilities, or assisted living communities. We do
not want to watch our loved ones decline, and we often are unprepared
to care for them when they can no longer care for themselves. Instead,
when they become sick, elderly, or frail we place them in institutions.
This is rarely an easy choice. But the ideal solution, if there is such a
thing, is not always available or affordable.

We commit Mom or Dad or Grandma or Grandpa to others' care
only after we have run out of other options. For instance, even if they
are willing to have a live-in caregiver, they may not be able to afford
it. We may be willing to take them into our homes but do not have
sufficient space to accommodate them. Perhaps we have children or
other dependents living with us and our primary responsibility is to care
for them. Or we may be one of the millions of American households
in which all the adults hold full-time jobs, making it impossible to stay
home during the day to care for an aged or ailing family member. We
may have a spouse or partner who objects to such an arrangement.

When it comes to rescuing our vulnerable loved ones from medical exile, there are an infinite number of obstacles.

If we do end up solving the problem by institutionalizing them, they are likely to face a set of problems at least as significant as the medical issues that caused them to be put there in the first place. Numerous studies have shown, for example, that sick, frail, or elderly individuals who are institutionalized often feel lonely, isolated, and bereft of dignity and autonomy.[1] The medical facility sets their daily schedule, limits their possessions, decides when they take their medicines, and in general dictates their daily life. They are safe but miserable—cut off from family and freedom. To all but a handful of people—the individuals charged with their care and the friends or family members who may visit them—they effectively cease to exist.

Joseph E. Davis, research professor of sociology at the University of Virginia, addresses this issue in an article titled "No Country for Old Age," noting that Americans seem to "regard aging and death as realities to hide."[2] Why can't we cope with our inevitable decline?" he asks rhetorically. "And why can't we maintain our sense of self in the face of dependency, disability, and an aging body?"

There is no simple answer to these cultural questions, which are discussed in some detail in chapter 3 of this book. However, Thomas R. Cole and Mary G. Winkler, editors of *The Oxford Book of Aging*, suggest that Americans are not the only ones who struggle with accepting old age, physical decline, and death. According to these scholars, "Western culture [collectively] offers few convincing ways to make sense of physical decline and the inevitability of death. For the most part, physical decay and death are still culturally construed as personal or medical failures, devoid of social or cosmic meaning."[3]

One need not be a social scientist to conclude that a culture that sees growing old and dying as failure is not going to bring happiness and contentment to America's seniors. Clearly, growing old and infirm and then dying is hard enough without being branded a failure as well. While no one has ever survived the GR, our society remains stubbornly irrational about the realities of death.

The good news is you can reject this nihilistic view of human frailty and set your own agenda for the balance of your days. What sort of life do you envision for yourself in the winter of your years, a stage of life that gerontologist Louise Aronson aptly terms "elderhood"? Sooner or later you will need to take ownership of that vision and of the some-times-difficult choices you will need to make in elderhood. Evidence shows that having a plan for elderhood, which for many truly becomes their golden years but in which we also are more likely to develop a chronic illness, is the key to both a happier life and a good death.

Now let's take a closer look at the choices we face at the end of life.

CHANGING SEASONS

"To every thing there is a season"—we read in *Ecclesiastes*, words written more than six thousand years ago—"and a time to every purpose under heaven."[4]

What, one might ask, is the purpose of growing old? Again, there are as many responses to this question as there are human beings who have lived long enough to experience both the wisdom and the deficits of age. One particularly wise perspective, I believe, was voiced by the great Roman statesman, lawyer, and philosopher Cicero, who lived in the first century BC. "Nature has fashioned human life so that we enjoy certain things when we are young and others when we are older," Cicero wrote in a book titled *How to Grow Old*.[5] "Attempting to cling to youth after the appropriate time is useless. If you fight nature, you will lose."[6]

Cicero also saw strengths and blessings in old age. Older people, he suggested, have much to teach the young. Wisdom can be gained only by experience. It is our pleasure and duty as we grow older to pass on that wisdom. According to Cicero, youths will teach their elders in this process as well. Humility and enlightenment go hand in hand.

Like many modern medical researchers, this most revered of all Roman philosophers believed that the mind is a muscle that must be exercised. It is vital to use our minds as much as possible as we grow older, he asserted. He also advised the elderly to cultivate their own garden, whether literally or figuratively. He believed that finding a worthwhile activity in our later years that gives true enjoyment is essential for happiness.

Cicero also stressed the importance of standing up for your dignity and expressing your beliefs regardless of your age. "Old age," he cautioned, "is respected only if it defends itself, maintains its rights, submits to no one, and rules over its domain until its last breath."[7]

Obviously, there were no nursing homes in Cicero's day and thus no chance for an aging patrician such as him to experience the dehumanizing losses associated with being institutionalized. One can only imagine the hell such a man would have raised if someone had attempted to commit him against his will to the Roman equivalent of a nursing home. (I encourage you to keep this in mind if you ever find yourself in a similar predicament.)

Death is not to be feared, declared Cicero. He suggested that death marks either the end of human consciousness or the beginning of eternal happiness. Or perhaps both. His death at age sixty-three in the year 43 BC was swift and dramatic. He was executed by assassins dispatched by Roman emperor Mark Antony, whom he had openly defied. He died courageously defending his beliefs. Today he is considered the greatest of the Roman philosophers, a man whose writings inspired the Western intellectual renaissance seventeen centuries later and whom Thomas Jefferson, a Founding Father, credited with inspiring some of the ideas of a "just republic" that are enshrined in the Declaration of Independence.[8]

BEING VS. DOING

When it comes to successfully navigating elderhood, attitude is everything. Put simply, how we think about old age will determine how we experience it. Like Cicero, we can graciously accept our inevitable losses and embrace the special joys and virtues of senior citizenship. We can stay engaged in the world, as he did, through relationships and meaningful pursuits. Or we can pretend that we're still young or spend our energy mourning our lost youth and wishing that our life circumstances were different. But wishing, hoping, or thinking won't solve the basic problem of being an aging human being. Nothing can change that. However, we can spare ourselves much angst and regret by adjusting the way in which we view ourselves.

Perhaps the hardest thing to let go of is our perception of ourselves as active players in the world, people with a mission in life that involves getting things done, things like making a living, building a career, choosing a life partner, raising a family, leaving our mark on the world. Who wants to become irrelevant? Who wants to be counted out of the active game of life and become a mere spectator? A geezer spectator at that!

Arthur C. Brooks, former CEO of the American Enterprise Institute, addressed this issue. "Decline is inevitable," wrote Brooks, "and it occurs earlier than almost all of us want to believe."[9] On the other hand, he posits, "misery is not inevitable. Accepting the natural cadence of our abilities sets up the possibility of transcendence, because it allows the shifting of attention to higher spiritual priorities."[10]

Brooks illustrates this point using two famous historical figures, the seventeenth-century German composer and musician Johann Sebastian Bach and the nineteenth-century English naturalist, geologist, and biologist Charles Darwin, whose theory of the evolution of species fundamentally changed how we see the world and our place in it. Both men had amazing success at a very young age. According to Brooks, both of these extraordinary individuals also experienced major setbacks in the middle of their lives.[11] When Darwin fell behind as an innovator, wrote Brooks, he became despondent and his life ended in sad inactivity. When Bach's musical creativity waned, he reinvented himself as a teacher and died beloved, fulfilled, and respected.

A REVERSE BUCKET LIST

Brooks notes in his article that as we age, our gifts and talents change. He suggests that like Bach we focus on developing new talents. He also confesses that with regard to his own personal status as a retired senior, "what I need to do . . . is stop seeing my life as a canvas to fill, and start seeing myself as a block of marble to chip away at and shape something out of. I need a reverse bucket list. My goal each year of the rest of my life should be to throw out things, obligations, and relationships until I can see my redefined self in its best form."[12]

I began following the path laid out by Arthur Brooks long before reading his article. I started ticking off items on my reverse bucket list soon after stepping down as CEO of Mercy Health (today Bon Secours Mercy), a large Catholic healthcare ministry owning and operating hospitals and clinics and serving thousands of patients in multiple states. At the time I stepped down, I was responsible for running a system that included over a thousand medical facilities and thirty hospitals with more than thirty-five thousand employees. Overnight my role changed from the leader of a large organization whose patients quite often depended on our employees to keep them alive to a retired citizen. The transition to being a retiree with no official duties or responsibilities was not a natural one. Although I had made the decision to step down voluntarily, I missed the daily challenges of being a chief executive, a role that had defined, even dominated, my life for the previous four decades. I was fortunate to become CEO of St. Joseph Hospital in Chicago at the age of thirty-two. That is a long time to be a CEO. Giving up my post also meant that I was no longer actively engaged in a helping profession, which was the reason I chose to work in the healthcare field. How do you replace your central purpose in life? How do you create a new identity?

I struggled with these issues but more at the outset than now, six years later. On the other hand, a great deal of stress was lifted off my shoulders when I retired, and frankly that felt—and still feels— exceptionally good. I have a sense of freedom that I have not felt since childhood. For most of my life I needed to focus all my energy on my obligations: supporting my family, raising the two sons and a daughter with whom my wife Sally and I have been blessed, and staying on top in my profession. My focus, though not uncommon, was pretty narrow. There was little time in my busy regimen for friends and even less time to pursue other interests.

In the end stage of my life, however, I have far fewer obligations. When my grandson Malcolm calls me on the phone and challenges me to a long-distance video game, I can surrender my time willingly while knowing that I am certain to be crushed in intergalactic warfare. I can have the pleasure of helping my granddaughter Grace with her math homework. I can indulge my intellectual curiosity by reading. (I have read more than one hundred books about healthcare and the end of life while researching this one.) I can cultivate neglected friendships and forge new ones. I can contribute to the world in ways that have nothing to do with building a legacy. I can accept my humble new role in life and find contentment in the little things—things I never would have been able to enjoy had I not stepped off the professional bandwagon when I did.

And as I have indicated in this book, I have the added peace that comes from accepting my own mortality. Because I have done that, I can live without the debilitating fear of death and dying. I'm confident that I will die one day like everyone else, but I have prepared for it. I have created a will, an AHD, and an HCPA. Unless my stated wishes are ignored, I will die naturally, at home and surrounded by my loved ones, rather than in an ICU or a nursing home with my body invaded by feeding tubes and hooked up to a ventilator or a dialysis machine. I will not be consigned to the purgatory of medical institutionalization where the best I could hope for would be to slowly waste away, one failed body part at a time, out of sight and out of mind for the young and the healthy. I will not share the fate of too many frail, elderly, or gravely ill Americans: I will not disappear. If you follow the guidelines found in this book for avoiding the death trap, you won't either.

10

OPTIONS FOR END-OF-LIFE CARE

> Those who contemplate their aging, vulnerability, and
> mortality often live better lives and experience better
> deaths than those who don't.
>
> —Katy Butler, *The Art of Dying Well: A Practical Guide to*
> *a Good End of Life*

Most Americans know little about old age, death, and dying. Considering that death is one of life's most significant events, however, ignorance of it may be a mistake, particularly regarding EOL care. The more you know, the more likely you will be to navigate your twilight years and avoid the death trap successfully. This is the death literacy of the *Lancet* research I discussed in the introduction, and pursuing it was one of the researchers' key recommendations.

Unless you die abruptly, your death is likely to follow a long and continuous decline marked by chronic illness and diminishing mental competence. Unfortunately, medical treatment for the frail and elderly—here in the United States or in any other country—has limited value. Nevertheless, many patients will still seek such treatment. According to Dr. Joanne Lynn, an expert in geriatrics and public health, the disabled and frail elderly population in this country will double over the next fifteen years, putting a severe strain on our healthcare resources.[1] Eventually most of these people will live out their days in an institutional setting. Three out of ten Americans today will die in a nursing home.[2] Five out of ten will expire in a hospital, and half of them in an ICU, which was not intended to treat such patients.[3]

If you would prefer to die at home without being tied to tubes and machines, you will need to educate yourself about the pros and cons of major treatment choices. In planning for EOL care, you will have three main choices: curative care, palliative care, or hospice care.

CURATIVE CARE

If you want all that medicine has to offer, no planning or preparation is necessary. If you are gravely ill in an American hospital and have no living will, you will automatically be thrust into the EOL healthcare machine. Like the hapless assembly-line worker in *Modern Times*—Charlie Chaplin's masterful satire of the perils of industrialization—you will be ratcheted through the machine's internal workings. When it is done treating you, the machine will spit you out again. Unlike the silent movie character, however, who emerges from his nightmare journey ruffled but physically intact, you may not fare as well.

Under the curative care paradigm, physicians will use all available medical means to extend your physical existence regardless of the side effects. On the plus side, this treatment approach most likely will keep you alive longer than any other. If that is your goal, this should be your choice. But keep in mind that this more aggressive treatment approach could subject you to a multitude of invasive procedures such as surgery; insertion of fluid or medicine-bearing needles in your veins; running a feeding tube through your nose, down your throat, and into your stomach; putting you on kidney dialysis; hooking you up to a ventilator (which requires inserting a plastic breathing tube in your throat); and reviving you through CPR or defibrillation (in which your heart is shocked to get it beating again or to restore a normal rhythm).

While these medical procedures can temporarily lengthen your stay on earth, they also can—indeed they almost certainly will—increase your misery. You are likely to experience physical pain, mental disorientation, and emotional distress as your body shuts down one organ at a time. Entire books have been written about the suffering due to this country's default treatment of terminally ill patients.

Unfortunately, only a handful of individuals will emerge from this experience with their health miraculously restored, like Lazarus awakened from the dead by Jesus. For everyone else in this predicament, the journey to the other side is likely to be cold and mechanized.

PALLIATIVE CARE

Palliative care, also known as comfort care or compassionate care, whether provided in a medical facility, such as a hospital or nursing home, or at your home, focuses on reducing your pain and boosting your quality of life. This is in contrast to prolonging your life, perhaps painfully, through medical intervention.

According to America's premier medical research organization, the National Institutes of Health (NIH):

> The goal of palliative care is to help people with serious illnesses feel better. It prevents or treats symptoms and side effects of disease and [medical] treatment. Palliative care also treats emotional, social, practical, and spiritual problems that illnesses can bring up. When the person feels better in these areas, they have an improved quality of life.[4]

Admittedly this definition is a mouthful, but it is accurate and comprehensive. The NIH also notes the key difference between palliative care and hospice care: "Both palliative care and hospice care provide comfort. But palliative care can begin at diagnosis, and at the same time as treatment."[5]

Palliative care allows for the option of curative care, and hospice does not allow for curative care. The distinct being that hospice is both an insurance product and a care model. Palliative care is only a care model.

"So Hospice care (see below) begins after treatment of the disease is stopped and when it is clear that the person is not going to survive the illness."[6]

Palliative care is comprehensive in nature. It can be provided to you by a host of healers ranging from palliative-care physicians to massage therapists to chaplains and psychologists. The goal is to treat the whole person and to address any area in which you might need comfort and support. For example, palliative treatment might include a counseling session with you and your family conducted by a social worker to assess your most pressing physical and emotional needs and to discuss possible solutions. You can receive palliative care at home as well as in a hospital, nursing home, or assisted living facility.

There are barriers to choosing palliative care. For one thing, it is difficult to access. Unlike hospice care, which services are covered by Medicare, palliative care has limited coverage from medical insurers. If you have Medicare Part B or Medicaid insurance, you may be reimbursed for some palliative-care services. However you will need to check with your insurer to learn which services are covered. The other reality is that palliative-care services, particularly in an outpatient setting, are difficult to find in today's health system.

A conceptual way to think about palliative care is to consider it at three different moments. The first moment would be as soon as you have been diagnosed with a terminal illness like advanced stage cancer or kidney failure. You understand that there are treatment options available for you, but you decide that the journey of the treatment is worse than the potential benefits of treatment and you choose to go into palliative care immediately. Or second, perhaps you decide to try a treatment therapy like chemotherapy or dialysis but after a few weeks conclude it isn't worth it and then go into palliative care. Third, you might exhaust your treatment options and then select palliative care at the very end, which at that stage would include hospice.

HOSPICE CARE

Modern hospice care, which originated in England during the 1960s, is a specific type of palliative medicine for people who have six months or less to live and who have stopped treatment for their condition. It is both a care model and an insurance product. Dame Cecily Sanders, the English doctor who first developed this care regimen to focus solely on the needs of the gravely ill or dying, summed up the essence of this now well-established branch of medicine in this way: "You matter because of who you are. You matter to the last moment of your life, and we will do all we can, not only to help you die peacefully, but also to live until you die."[7]

In the United States, hospice care is widely available but often it is not pursued as a care option until the patient is just days away from dying. This is certainly understandable—who wants to contemplate their own death? However, countless research studies have shown that people who enroll in hospice before their illness turns critical report a much higher quality of life in their remaining days than those who wait until the last minute to sign up.[8]

Hospice provides the same range of services you would receive via palliative care with two differences: (1) You will receive no curative treatment for your underlying illness; (2) Your hospice care will not also support your family. The goal of hospice care is to allow you to experience a natural death, a death as free of pain and distress as can humanly be made possible. If hospice is your EOL care preference, you can set this up directly with a hospice provider or you can ask your physician to arrange it.

Most U.S. communities have more than one hospice option. To qualify for hospice insurance coverage, two independent physicians must certify that you are likely to die within the next six months based on the usual course of your disease. Usually the hospice itself will obtain these physician approvals once it has assessed your health status.

As simple as this process may sound, however, you may find yourself in an uphill battle to obtain hospice care. Physicians by training and by virtue of the American healthcare system's bias toward curative medicine are often reluctant to refer a patient to hospice. Making such a referral requires your doctor to admit that they have failed to save your life. You also may face resistance from family members who are not ready to accept that you are dying. Your family may encourage you to fight to the last breath to stay alive. Neither of these well-intended interlocutors, however, will be doing you any favors by artificially lengthening your life—or viewed another way, by extending the dying process.

This quandary is eloquently summed up by hospice volunteer Katy Butler. She personalizes the issue by describing her own preferences for EOL care. "My wish is to die in my own bed," she says, "cared for by people I love—clean, comfortable and relatively free from pain. I hope I have time to say my goodbyes and give my final blessings."[9]

Hard to achieve? Yes, but not impossible. In fact, you can clearly express your preference for palliative care, including hospice and a natural death, by executing an AHD. This legal document will allow you to spell out the type and the limits of the healthcare you wish to receive at the end of your days. (AHDs along with HCPAs will be discussed in greater detail in chapter 11.)

Perhaps the most telling thing you will learn in exploring EOL care options is that an informed patient frequently chooses palliative care, including hospice, over curative care. For example, most physicians take this path for their own care. As an informed healthcare consumer, I came to the same conclusion independently. Based on what I saw and learned while working in the healthcare field for more than four decades, I believe palliative care is the most humane, dignified, and comprehensive EOL care option available. That is why I have requested this EOL paradigm for myself in my AHD. The key is knowing when to transition from curative care to compassion care.

ASSISTED SUICIDE

Though their numbers are still relatively small, some terminally ill Americans are choosing assisted suicide as a way to end their suffering. Though assisted suicide is not a treatment option per se, I'm including this controversial practice in this chapter since it relates to the end of life. Under this medical paradigm, a physician enables you to actively induce your own death by prescribing a lethal dose of a barbiturate or other sedative drug. The final decision on whether or not to swallow the pills is up to you—the patient.

This practice is more prevalent in other countries, most notably the Netherlands, which has, basically, removed all legal penalties for physician-assisted suicide. Americans, by contrast, have been generally more reluctant to allow doctors to help them hasten their demise. Currently ten U.S. states and the District of Columbia have legally authorized physicians to assist terminally ill patients in dying. In the remaining forty states, helping someone die is illegal and can be prosecuted as a crime.

The so-called death-with-dignity laws that were enacted have built-in safeguards requiring both the doctor and the patient contemplating assisted suicide to respond to a series of screens aimed at preventing impulsive decision-making by the patient. It is worth noting that following this mandatory review process, reportedly only about one out of ten patients who had planned to induce their own death actually followed through with it.[10]

Sadly, the movement for assisted suicide is symptomatic of a healthcare system that is not effectively responding to patient concerns at end of life. If patients had broader access to palliative care, virtually all their concerns and fears could be addressed without their resorting to suicide. The inability of patients to have meaningful conversations with their caregivers to address these fears is at the core of this issue.

Due to my faith I would not choose assisted suicide for myself. Regarding my beliefs, I know that I did not bring myself into this world, and I am content to entrust the timing of my exit to the same higher power that decided when I would be born. However, presuming to judge others on this matter is beyond my comfort level. As Pope Francis notes in *The Name of God is Mercy*, "Who am I to judge?"[11] But as the English writer G. K. Chesterton also observed, "Art, like morality, consists of drawing the line somewhere."[12]

HELPING YOU CHOOSE

As medical science advances, EOL care choices will become even more complex and challenging. I believe the best way to sort through your options is a discussion with your primary care physician (PCP) or nurse practitioner who has been trained in palliative care. No one else knows you and your medical history as well or is in a better position to advise you on this sensitive topic. Unfortunately this may be hollow advice because few primary care practices are prepared to have this conversation. But regardless of where you seek advice (and advice is important), you can begin exploring your preferences as part of your planning process.

One of the most helpful medical decision-making tools I have found is the benefit vs. burden analytical model. This simple, straightforward decision model, which originated in Catholic ethical teachings, involves a frank, personal assessment of what you can expect to gain and, conversely, what you can expect to lose when you face and make a difficult choice. In the case of EOL care, for example, you might ask yourself, "Will the additional time I might gain be worth the discomfort caused by the invasive medical interventions that will be required to keep me alive?" Obviously, this is a decision that only you can make.

To better understand this decision model, let's look at a medical issue that arises frequently at the end of life: the inability to eat or hold down food. One could argue that the best treatment for such a patient would be a feeding tube. Imagine for a moment you are that patient. This common procedure would provide you with the basic sustenance you needed to stay alive. But would extending your life for a limited time outweigh the discomfort of having a tube threaded through your nostrils, down your throat, and into your stomach or of having that feeding tube implanted directly in your stomach through a surgical incision? You also would need to ask yourself, "Will the feeding tube change or improve my underlying illness or merely buy me a little more time?"

Although miracles do happen, most patients with a feeding tube are not likely to recover. Nevertheless, some see a benefit in delaying death and are willing to accept the pain and suffering that will result from this medical intervention in return for extending their life. However, others facing the same harrowing choice will conclude that given their grave physical condition and the remote likelihood of ever returning to normal life activities, the burden of the feeding tube outweighs the benefits. A very good friend of mine who recently died made this choice.

KEVIN'S CHOICE

Kevin and I had been friends since we attended a Catholic elementary school together in a large midwestern city back in the early 1960s. When we later entered high school, Kevin was of modest physical stature so his participation in competitive team sports at our large, all-boys high school was not an option. However, Kevin found a way to display his dexterity and express his strong school spirit by becoming a cheerleader.

Amazingly, my former classmate grew six more inches during his senior year and another six inches while attending college. His girth also expanded. As an adult he stood six-feet-five inches tall and weighed nearly 290 pounds. As an adult, Kevin also developed chronic health problems, including borderline diabetes. At one point, he suffered pulmonary blood clots, which can be deadly. Both of his knees wore out and had to be replaced.

Despite his health problems, Kevin remained physically and socially active. Due to his personal charm, he excelled in his career in sales. Kevin also enjoyed social gambling. During our high school days, he hosted poker games at his parents' house. As an adult, he made several memorable trips to Las Vegas. His greatest gift was his ability to befriend people and to keep those friendships going. He developed close personal bonds with people from all walks of life. Some were millionaires. Others were homeless. All were equal in his eyes. Kevin was the kind of person who was willing to put in the time and work required to bring people together.

Kevin truly enjoyed playing golf, as did I and many of his other friends. Over the years he used our shared passion for the sport to bring us together. For forty-five consecutive years he was an active participant in a Father's Day weekend golf tournament that invariably drew twenty to thirty of us back to our hometown to hit the links, share memories of our youthful indiscretions, and rekindle old friendships. Kevin organized annual golf outings to Pebble Beach, Pinehurst, and Kiawah for a smaller group of us who went to grade school together. I happily participated in several of these gatherings later in life.

In 2018, Kevin convinced me and more than thirty other old friends to join him in celebrating his sixty-fifth birthday. It was a grand occasion, with Kevin relishing his role as the master of ceremonies at this party he had arranged for his friends. The gathering was far more than a birthday celebration, however. It marked the joyful renewal of a lifelong bond among a group of senior citizens who had met as schoolboys nearly half a century ago. None of us suspected that we were about to lose the glue that had held us all together for so many years.

Like so many other life-changing events, Kevin's final undoing was both unexpected and mundane. He tripped on the stairs while carrying a basket of dirty clothes down to his basement laundry room. He suffered damage to his vertebrae so severe it left him paralyzed from the neck down. He underwent back surgery. He was placed in a nursing home, where he tried to rehabilitate himself in hopes of recovering at least some movement in his arms or legs. Sadly, his effort failed. As happens frequently to bedridden, immobilized patients, he developed blood clots in his lungs. He made two emergency trips to the hospital where he was successfully treated for this condition. But Kevin could see the writing on the wall. Spending the rest of his days in a nursing home and completely dependent on others for the basic functions of life was not a viable option for this energetic, outgoing man. At the same time, burdening his family with the personal and financial demands of such an existence seemed not just unfair to Kevin, it was unthinkable. My sixty-seven-year-old friend was facing the greatest dilemma of his life.

Kevin's medical crisis came to a head when he began throwing up virtually everything he ate. Unfortunately, additional gastrointestinal treatment and testing failed to alleviate the problem. The only way to avoid the pain caused by his involuntary retching was to stop eating—which Kevin did. If he wanted to stay alive, he would need a feeding tube.

After weighing the pros and cons of the proposed medical intervention, he decided that the benefit of gaining a little more time was not worth the burden of a feeding tube. He also faced a uniquely depressing reality brought on by the COVID-19 pandemic: to protect highly susceptible residents from infection, many nursing homes, such as Kevin's, imposed a total ban on visitors. For a man who had thrived on social contact, this was a spiritual death sentence. After fighting valiantly, but unsuccessfully, to recover from his injuries, Kevin decided it was time to end an unwinnable battle. He declined the feeding tube.

Around a week before Kevin died, he called me from the nursing home. He told me he was going into hospice care. Although it shouldn't have, his news caught me by surprise. I did not know what to say. I knew his decision had come after much suffering and that making it almost certainly was the hardest thing he had ever had to do. I believed he had made the right choice. If I did not believe this, I would be a hypocrite. After all, dying naturally is how I plan to go. Yet I felt uneasy telling Kevin that I supported his decision. In effect, my old friend was giving up, passively accepting death. How could I possibly approve of such an action? Would that not make me complicit in his demise? Was it not my duty as a friend to encourage Kevin to keep fighting?

In the United States, we are encouraged to fight injustice—and what greater injustice can there possibly be than losing your life? "Never give up" is the mantra of our culture. But in the endgame of life, fighting to the bitter end with everything you've got also can work against you. Clearly Kevin realized this, and he decided to use the precious moments he had left to say goodbye to the people he loved.

A few days after receiving Kevin's distressing phone call, I and two more of his closest friends decided we needed to say goodbye to him in person. Kevin's wife was kind enough to make special arrangements with the hospice and grant us permission to visit. When we entered Kevin's room, we found this amiable giant, who always had seemed larger than life to us, dozing. We were shocked by his appearance. He had lost much of his body weight. His skin was pallid and hung loosely on his oversized frame. He looked like a soldier would look after a long, bloody fight against an unforgiving enemy. We all took seats near his bed. When one of us gently spoke his name, he slowly opened his eyes. They lit up when he saw that we had made a special effort to visit him.

For the next two hours, we had a very moving experience. It was as if we had been magically transported back to the days when we were young, strong, and foolish. We joyfully relived our youthful misadventures together. We talked about our families, our golfing trips, the wonderful meals we had shared, and, of course, the parties. We openly expressed our love for Kevin. We thanked him for his countless efforts over the years to keep us united as a band of brothers. Shortly before taking our leave, we all gave Kevin a hug. Then every person in the room, including Kevin, broke down and cried.

In looking back on this unforgettable moment, my only regret is that I did not tell him how much I admired him for facing death head on. His decision was courageous and selfless. Unfortunately, I could not bring myself to acknowledge his bravery. Knowing Kevin, however, he has forgiven me.

11

PREPARING PAPERWORK FOR ELDERHOOD

By failing to prepare, you are preparing to fail.

—Benjamin Franklin

If your wish is to die naturally, the best way to ensure that outcome is to educate yourself about EOL care and then use that knowledge to execute an AHD and an HCPA. Putting these legally binding documents in place before your health starts to decline could mean the difference between comfort and misery.

An AHD spells out the type as well as the limits of the medical care you wish to receive at the end of your life. Its primary purpose is to inform your medical caregivers and healthcare surrogate of your treatment preferences should you reach the point where you can no longer make decisions for yourself due to illness or mental incapacity. However, as aptly noted by medical attorney Amanda Singleton, there are other compelling reasons for creating an advance directive. For example, an AHD can allow you to "provide clarity and closure to your loved ones, prevent conflict or disagreements among family members, and limit the emotional burden on your closest people at the time of your death."[1]

Ms. Singleton said she considered her own mother's decision to create an advance directive a gift to both of them. She said her mother learned about her EOL treatment options, decided which of them she did and did not want to receive, then made sure her preferences were clearly spelled out in her advance directive. Because her caregivers were aware of her advance directive and willing to honor it, Ms. Singleton's mother was able to die naturally, according to her wishes.

"All I had to do was be a daughter. To hold my mother's hand, sing and talk to her, and wait. And when she passed away, my heart, mind and soul were at peace."[2]

One of the factors contributing to Ms. Singleton's peace of mind was her knowledge, as an attorney, that her mother's living will was not just a piece of paper with instructions written on it. It was an official document with clear instructions of her preferences. In recent years, some physicians have pursued a model of care called advanced care planning (ACP). This is the practice of planning with patients and their family how they wish to receive care near the end of their life. ACP is a wonderful foundational tool for completing one's AHD. In this country, healthcare providers are bound to honor the stated wishes of a properly executed AHD—assuming they are aware of the document!

HISTORY AND ORIGINS

According to recent national surveys, only three out of ten Americans have an AHD in place.[3] Unfortunately just checking the boxes to complete these documents is not adequate. As discussed above, you need to fully understand the documents you are completing. Unfortunately, most model directives offer an option to indicate that you don't want "extraordinary care." This statement may in your mind seem to protect you from futile care. Unfortunately it doesn't work out that way. The term "extraordinary care" is ambiguous and subject to different interpretations, making it virtually useless as guidance to caregivers and families because it has no meaningful definition. What is needed are more precise statements like "No ventilator" or "No dialysis" or "No feeding tubes" or "I would like to die at home." These statements are the types of instructions that are useful to decision makers. If you go through the ACP process with your physician, making these choices is easier. But ACPs are not a widely used practice because they are not generally supported economically or clinically.

Of the 70 percent of Americans without an AHD, most know little or nothing about these medical planning documents even though they have been available in the United States for more than half a century. In 1967, Chicago human rights lawyer Luis Kutner reportedly drafted the first living will after watching the torturous hospital death of a close friend following a long and painful illness. Kutner believed his friend suffered needlessly during his final days due to the fruitless medical interventions used to keep him alive, and he wanted to protect others from suffering a similar fate.

The novel concept of protecting a dying patient from the excesses of well-meaning but overzealous healers caught on slowly. Nine years later in 1976, California became the first state to legally sanction living wills. A handful of other states gradually followed suit, but it was not until 1990 that the terms "living will" and "advance healthcare directive" became part of the national lexicon. That was the year in which the U.S. Supreme Court ruled on its first right-to-die case.

CRUZAN V. DIRECTOR, MISSOURI DEPARTMENT OF HEALTH

On January 11, 1983, twenty-five-year-old Nancy Cruzan lost control of her car while driving home late at night from her job at a cheese factory near Carthage, Missouri. She was thrown from her vehicle and landed face-down in a water-filled ditch. By the time paramedics arrived, she had stopped breathing. They managed to revive her, but she had been deprived of oxygen for so long she suffered irreversible brain damage. She was comatose when admitted to the hospital. Three weeks later, her doctors concluded she was in a persistent vegetative state, meaning she had no brain function and virtually no hope of recovery. She could breathe on her own but could not eat or control any of her bodily functions. Surgeons inserted a feeding tube into her stomach to keep her alive.

The cruelty of the young woman's plight was made clear when a writer allegedly described her rigid body with feet and hands contracted and bent. Reportedly she had occasional seizures and vomited, and her eyes sometimes opened and moved though she showed no sign of recognizing her family.

Four years later, Nancy's grief-stricken parents, Lester and Joyce Cruzan, decided their daughter had suffered long enough. They asked her doctors to remove her feeding tube to allow her to die. However, the hospital refused. Her parents went to court. They won their first legal battle when a trial court ruled that Nancy Cruzan had effectively directed the withdrawal of life support by telling a friend earlier that year that if she were sick or injured, "she would not wish to continue her life unless she could live at least halfway normally."

However, the State of Missouri appealed the ruling to the Missouri Supreme Court and won. Nancy Cruzan's parents fought that ruling all the way to the U.S. Supreme Court, which heard the opposing arguments on their daughter's right to die on December 6, 1989. The following June, the justices ruled 5-4 to uphold the ruling by the Missouri Supreme Court that Lester and Joyce Cruzan had failed to provide clear and convincing evidence that their daughter would elect to have her feeding tube removed if she were able to speak. Apparently, they dismissed the trial testimony given by the friend of Nancy Cruzan who said Nancy had told her she would not want to continue to live in a severely compromised state. And they gave no legal weight to her parents' rights or wishes.

According to legal analysts, the key precedent set by the Supreme Court ruling was that only one person can legally decide whether to accept or reject medical treatment, and that person is *you.*[4] If you cannot speak for yourself but have a living will, the preferences you spelled out in that document must be followed. If there is no such document, the burden then falls on your family to provide clear and convincing evidence of what you would choose.[5] Absent such evidence, the Supreme Court ruled, the decision on whether or not to continue life support must be made by the state in which the patient resides. In effect, the court agreed with the State of Missouri that it had the right and the duty to protect Nancy Cruzan from being put to death by her parents by removing her feeding tube.

Having established its authority to decide life-or-death medical issues being faced by Missouri residents, the State of Missouri withdrew from the case. Lester and Joyce Cruzan again petitioned a local court for the right to remove their daughter's feeding tube. At that November 1990 hearing, former coworkers of Nancy Cruzan recalled her saying she would never want to live "like a vegetable." Her doctor described her existence as a "living hell" and said her feeding tube should be removed.

This time the state chose not to intervene, and the family's request was granted. This lower court concluded clear and convincing evidence was provided during this trial. Doctors finally removed the device on December 14, 1990, nearly eight years after Nancy Cruzan had been thrown from her car. Four days later, the already notorious case took another dramatic turn when a group of right-to-life proponents snuck into the hospital where Nancy Cruzan lay unconscious and tried to reattach her feeding tube. They failed, and all nineteen of them were arrested.

On December 26, the then thirty-three-year-old woman died. "Knowing Nancy as only a family can," her parents said in a formal statement to the press, "there remains no question that we made the choice she would want. She remained peaceful throughout and showed no sign of discomfort or distress."

At Nancy's funeral, her father told reporters, "I would prefer to have my daughter back and let someone else be this trailblazer [for the right to die without governmental interference]."[6] Six years later, Lester Cruzan killed himself, adding a new layer of sadness to this family's tragedy.

As is often true in human history, progress comes at a high cost. In addition to exposing one family's heartbreaking ordeal to the world, the Nancy Cruzan case brought unprecedented national attention to the legal and ethical questions surrounding the right to die. According to a report in the *New York Times*, the Supreme Court's controversial ruling "spurred enormous interest in living wills and other advance directives that allow people to spell out, in advance, what treatment they want, and who should make decisions for them if they become incapacitated."[7] In the month after the ruling, the newspaper noted, the Society for the Right to Die answered nearly 300,000 requests for advance directive forms.[8]

The *New York Times* also reported that the Nancy Cruzan case helped generate support for Congressional passage of the 1991 Patient Self-Determination Act "under which hospitals and nursing homes that receive Medicaid or Medicare funds must give patients written information about such advance directives, explaining what right-to-die options are available under their state law."[9] By 1992, just two years after Nancy Cruzan was removed from life support, all fifty U.S. states and the District of Columbia had passed legislation supporting advance directives.

I believe we owe a debt of gratitude to the Cruzan family for showing us how important it is to make your wishes known about how you would want to be treated—or not treated—should you suffer a fate similar to Nancy Cruzan's.

CREATING YOUR ADVANCE DIRECTIVE

Although there are slight variations from state to state, every U.S. state has an official advance directive form that is available on the Internet. In the State of South Carolina, where I live, the AHD form includes a page titled "Declaration of a Desire for a Natural Death." On that page, I am asked to confirm that I "willfully and voluntarily make known my desire that no life-sustaining procedures be used to prolong my dying if my condition is terminal or if I am in a state of permanent unconsciousness." I also am asked to specify which life-sustaining medical procedures I specifically reject; for example, using cardiopulmonary resuscitation or a defibrillator to shock me back to life if my heart stops. If I do not want this to happen, I must execute a Do Not Resuscitate (DNR) order. Likewise, if I don't want to be hooked up to a ventilator or a dialysis machine, receive antibiotics, or undergo surgery, I must specify these preferences as well. While filling out my advance directive, I checked all the boxes. Provided my wishes are honored, I will not be kept futilely alive through these or any other artificial means.

When you are ready to create your advance directive, try to make an appointment with your primary care physician (PCP) and request an advanced care planning session. Because your doctor knows you and your medical history, he or she will be best equipped to explain your EOL care options and to respond to any questions or concerns you might have. If for some reason your doctor is not comfortable with this request, ask for a referral to another healthcare professional such as a palliative-care physician or nurse, who specializes in EOL care.

Based on this conversation, you should make a list of the medical interventions you do and, even more importantly, *do not wish* to receive in your final days. Be specific. For example, if you were to slip into unconsciousness, would you want to continue receiving medication, food, and fluids intravenously? What if you were suffering from Alzheimer's or some other form of dementia and you no longer could feed yourself or recognize loved ones? Would you want your healthcare providers to keep your body going despite your negligible quality of life?

Admittedly these are bleak topics. But based on what I have learned during my four decades working in healthcare, I can assure you that dealing with them now is far preferable to allowing someone else, someone who may barely know you, to decide your medical fate when you are no longer able to do so yourself.

Before formalizing your wishes with an advance directive, it is important to discuss your preferences with your spouse or another close family member or friend.

YOUR ADVANCE DIRECTIVE AND ELECTRONIC MEDICAL RECORD

Offering patients the opportunity to complete their advance directive in their electronic record with their physician would be a wonderful strategy. Most electronic records have a patient portal where patients can log on and see their test results, history, and other helpful information. EPIC is the name of the largest electronic record in the United States, and it calls this portal MYCHART. My recommendation is that all electronic medical providers offer model advance directives in these patient portals. This practice would be standardized for all electronic records. Just as patients receive reminders to have vaccinations or other tests, patients would be reminded to complete an AHD. Having this document embedded in every electronic medical record would encourage patients and physicians to have a conversation about the importance of an AHD and how each person should choose to complete one.

A second electronic record strategy would be to enhance the accessibility of any AHD because clinicians often claim they are difficult to locate. A variety of approaches would achieve this improved accessibility. For example, records for patients over age sixty-five could have a prominent flag highlighting their AHD. My primary concern is that clinicians don't naturally think about EOL care, and making any patient's AHD more visible and accessible helps address the issue.

A third and more sophisticated strategy would be to use an embedded and completed AHD to flag contraindicated care. For instance, if a patient has specified they do not want a feeding tube and one is ordered for the patient, the chart would flag that order as contraindicated. Software in the record is designed to do this flagging for medications. A similar technique could be used for management of EOL care. This would be the ultimate integration of the AHD and the electronic record.

Facilitating these conversations on EOL care is unlikely in the current healthcare system. However, in chapters 12 and 13, I recommend changes in the delivery system that might encourage these conversations. A more supportive electronic record would be another nudge to move healthcare in this direction.

HEALTHCARE POWER OF ATTORNEY

If you want to increase the likelihood that your EOL care preferences will be honored, you should also execute a HCPA. This legal document authorizes an individual chosen by you to make EOL medical decisions for you should you become mentally or physically incapacitated. Rather than depending solely on a document to ensure that your wishes are honored, you essentially are making a known individual responsible for your medical care.

There is no hard-and-fast rule regarding whom you should select as your medical surrogate, but here are some criteria you could use to narrow down your list.

- Does this person know you well and know how you feel about EOL care?
- Will they have the time and be available to communicate with your caregivers when needed?
- Is this person knowledgeable about healthcare issues and comfortable discussing them?
- Will they be objective enough under stress to make difficult decisions on your behalf?

The purpose of these questions is to help you select the best-qualified person to assume this important responsibility on your behalf.

PHYSICIAN ORDERS FOR LIFE-SUSTAINING TREATMENT

Physician orders for life-sustaining treatment (POLST) are a distinct approach to EOL care where physicians discuss with their severely ill patients specific medical orders to be honored by healthcare workers during a medical crisis. It differs from your advance directive in that it is a physician order not a patient order and therefore must be followed by all caregivers. So for example, a patient in hospice at home falls and a caregiver calls 911. The patient needs help but does not wish to go to the hospital. Usually the paramedics would be required to take that patient to the hospital, but a POLST order could override that obligation and force the paramedics to stabilize the patient at home.

The use of these orders requires state-law authorization. The concept started in 1991 in Oregon, and today forty-six states have authorized these orders for physicians. Essentially these orders document what type of care a patient does *not* want to receive. It is an attempt to limit the death trap.

The POLST document is a standardized, mobile (treatment is not location specific), brightly colored, single-page medical order that documents a conversation between the physician and an individual with a serious illness near the end of life.

It is important to emphasize that a POLST form is not a substitute for an advance directive—it is meant to complement it.

The POLST represents a healthcare policy by which provider communication is standardized through a care plan that is mobile. It begins with a conversation between the healthcare professional and the individual (or the individual's surrogate) about treatment options in light of the individual's current condition. The individual's preferences for treatment determine the nature of the medical orders. For instance, these orders may specify the level of intervention desired in an emergency such as comfort care or the use of artificial nutrition and hydration or the use of a ventilator. One of the primary drivers for the POLST initiative was fragmented healthcare. These mobile orders ensure consistent communication among all caregivers regardless of location.

IMPLEMENTING YOUR WISHES

Once you have completed your AHD and HCPA, these documents will need to be entered in your electronic medical record so they will be available to those caring for you. As long as you remain mentally competent, you can amend your advance directive or HCPA at any time. Every few years, or if your health status changes, you will want to review these documents with your physician and medical surrogate to make sure the documents reflect your current thinking on how you wish to receive EOL care and whom you wish to empower to oversee your care.

In my view, having an AHD and a HCPA in place is even more important than having a last will and testament for your estate. While many people may not have significant assets to distribute, everyone has human dignity, and no one wants to suffer unnecessarily. Preserving your dignity and protecting yourself from needless suffering is worth investing the time and effort required to put your plan into place.

Please keep in mind that you will not be the sole beneficiary of such planning. Creating a clear blueprint for your EOL care will relieve your loved ones of having to make complex, life-and-death medical decisions they may be ill-equipped or reluctant to make. Believe me, they will be stressed out enough by the thought of losing you without having this added burden placed on them. In fact, recently the daughter of a dying mother told me she was distressed and offended when she was asked to make an EOL care decision by her mother's doctors.

CHANGING YOUR MIND

When death comes, how will you react? Will you be brave, steadfast, and firm? Or will you panic at the first sign of impending mortality? After all, it's not uncommon for people to change their mind when the big moment finally arrives.

We're only human, and how we thought we'd deal with death in theory can quickly change in practice. Undoubtedly fear and uncertainty of the unknown can make it hard to complete an advance directive with confidence. The simple truth is it's difficult to make decisions about emotionally laden events because it's impossible to truly know how we'll feel at that moment.

There is no cure-all for this problem of emotional uncertainty, but there are ways to prepare. For instance, education and reflection are invaluable assets in terms of making wise, informed choices. Education-wise, a more thorough understanding of the implications of EOL care treatment should give you more confidence. Similarly, some proactive reflection on the question "When am I old enough to die?" can potentially prevent you from panicking and seeking desperate options to stay alive.

Finally, you might take some solace from reflecting on how physicians make decisions like these for themselves. Physicians, arguably, are the most educated and prepared individuals to make EOL care decisions. Numerous studies demonstrate that physicians are minimalists when it comes to seeking curative care for themselves at the end of life. Their education on these issues gives them confidence to make these decisions.

While all the preparation in the world cannot ensure a peaceful death or stop someone from changing their mind at a crucial moment, lack of preparation is a recipe for chaos. As such, developing your death literacy on the issues surrounding EOL care will improve your understanding and confidence in preparing your advance directive.

IF YOU HELP THEM, THEY WILL PLAN

In 1986, Dr. Bernard Hammes, at the time a clinical ethicist at a large, nonprofit healthcare system based in La Crosse, Wisconsin, set up a novel patient education program that showed how quickly people embrace medical planning if they are offered incentives. Clinical patients at the Gundersen Health System—which operates hospitals, clinics, and a large health insurance plan in Wisconsin, Minnesota, and Iowa—were given the chance to discuss their EOL care options with their doctor. Then specially trained nurses, chaplains, and social workers were employed by the health system to help these patients complete advance directive and HCPA forms.

The results of this experiment, which since has morphed into an internationally renowned patient education program called Respecting Choices, have been remarkable. When the EOL planning first was offered, more than eight out of ten elderly patients receiving healthcare services from the Gundersen Health System signed up.[10] And the enthusiasm didn't stop there. By 1996, 96 percent of the 540 adult La Crosse residents who had died in the previous year had an advance directive in place to guide their medical caregivers.[11] This was nearly three times the national average of people with an AHD and the highest percentage of any city in the world.

Why was the AHD adoption rate so high among Gundersen patients and what were the results? By being allowed to complete their advance directive in their physician's office, the patients were more likely to be informed about their choices and their caregivers to better understand those choices. As a result, patients in the Gundersen Health System were far more likely than typical patients to receive the care they desired at the end of life.

The reason for the program's popularity is no great mystery. It appears that most people will jump at the chance to learn more about what to expect at the end of life and to decide in advance what sort of medical care they will receive—especially if the counseling is offered free of charge as it was by Gundersen. The health system, on the other hand, will spend millions of dollars each year compensating its staff members for the professional time they devote to counseling patients.

"We just built it into the overhead of the organization," explains Dr. Hammes, who later left Gundersen Health to set up an organization to help other health systems, hospitals, and clinics implement and adapt the Respecting Choices educational model to their particular system.[12] "We believe it's part of good patient care. We believe that our patients deserve to have an opportunity to have these conversations."[13]

Though the program is costly to administer, since Gundersen owns a large health insurance plan, the savings from avoiding unnecessary EOL care provides a source of funding for this innovative counseling program. Arguably Gundersen is offering its patients something no amount of money can buy: a chance to take the mystery and fear out of the dying process by talking with a person who understands the complexities of EOL care and is willing to walk them through the decision-making process with empathy and emotional support. However, as Dr. Hammes stressed in a 2014 interview, "the ultimate content of this conversation, I think, isn't about death. I think the ultimate topic that's being discussed is how people care for each other. And so, what comes out at the end of the conversation is 'I love you, and I now know how to take good care of you.'"[14]

Dr. Hammes said he realized, soon after assuming his professional duties at Gundersen in 1984, which included counseling families of gravely ill patients, how helpful these conversations could be. "When I asked these family members [who had asked for his help], 'What would your dad want, what would your mom want, what did they say to you previously?' The response was the same again and again. The response was 'If only I knew.'"[15]

The medical ethicist acknowledged that after counseling numerous patients and their families about EOL care, he realized that just handing them the paperwork for an advance directive rarely produced any beneficial results. Few of them filled out the form. Offering to sit down with the patients to personally answer their questions and address their fears, on the other hand, and then helping them formalize their wishes in a written plan, Dr. Hammes found, made all the difference in the world. Hence, the creation of Respecting Choices.

Today the patient education model developed by Dr. Hammes and some of his professional colleagues at Gundersen Health is being used by more than 150 American medical centers as well as by hospitals, clinics, and health systems in Singapore, Australia, and Germany. Six other European Union countries—Belgium, Denmark, Italy, the Netherlands, Slovakia, and the United Kingdom—are researching the program and are expected to adopt it as well.

Giving more people the chance to plan their EOL medical care, it turns out, also can save money—lots of it, in fact. Per capita, Medicare spending on Gundersen Health System patients with advance directives in their last two years of life consistently runs 40 percent below the national average.[16]

If every hospital, clinic, and health system in America offered its patients free EOL care counseling and help in filling out their planning documents, Medicare spending on EOL care, which adds up to billions of dollars each year, would be reduced dramatically. And countless more Americans would be spared from undergoing invasive medical procedures that cannot save their lives.

12

UNDERSTANDING THE FFS PHYSICIAN PAYMENT SYSTEM

> I look at the U.S. healthcare system and see an administrative monstrosity, a genuinely bizarre mélange of thousands of payers with payment systems that differ for no socially beneficial reason, as well as staggeringly complex public systems with mind-boggling administered prices and other rules expressing distinctions that can only be described as weird.
>
> —Henry Aaron, economist, writing in the *New England Journal of Medicine*

If we want to change EOL care in America, we need to start by reforming the so-called fee for service (FFS) healthcare payment model. If you want to know why physicians don't have adequate time to talk with their patients, the answer is the FFS model. This antiquated, highly inefficient financial structure dates back to the passage of Medicare in 1965. Before Medicare, physicians were free to bill patients according to their preferences. In those days, most physicians were in primary care practices. That all changed with Medicare. This healthcare insurance program for seniors was built on a physician fee schedule that paid doctors a standard, predetermined fee for providing a specific medical service to a patient such as a blood test, x-ray, or injection. These standard fees did not recognize differences in quality or the physician's experience level and depended heavily on the concept that all care could be measured. This insurance payment program quickly became the dominant player in the healthcare marketplace because of Medicare's growing influence on the insurance market. The entire American healthcare system eventually adopted Medicare's FFS model.

Unhappily, what started out as a relatively simple and straightforward system has evolved into a financial and bureaucratic nightmare due to an explosion of complexity in the coding system that drives this payment model. Health insurers use two coding systems: the Current Procedural Terminology (CPT) system, created and maintained by the American Medical Association, and the International Statistical Classification of Diseases and Related Health Problems (ICD), under the keeping of the World Health Organization. ICD codes are focused on diagnoses while CPT codes describe the medical services or procedures undertaken to address the diagnosed injury or disease. The ICD codes determine the CPT code for billing.

Today, incredibly, there are more than 70,000 procedure (CPT) codes and 69,000 diagnostic (ICD) codes! The latter include Y92.253—*Hurt at the Opera*; W55.21—*Bitten by a Cow*; and V91.07XA—*Burn Due to Water Skis on Fire*. These codes may seem absurd, but they are legitimate. It is the CPT codes, however, that are used to report procedures and services to federal and private insurers so they can calculate payments to physicians for the rendered services. Adding a new layer of complexity to the process, the insurers then assign a relative value unit, or RVU, to each CPT code based on its complexity when compared with similar procedures or services. For example, Code 69209, *Remove impacted ear wax unilaterally,* is assigned 0.40 RVUs. But Code 69220, *Clean out mastoid cavity*, which is more extensive and involves more resources, gets 2.25 RVUs. And because of its far greater complexity, Code 69150, *Extensive ear canal surgery,* receives 29.25 RVUs.

Are you confused yet? Don't feel bad if you are. This labyrinthine system for determining FFS reimbursements confuses everyone. But wait, there's more. The dollar value of each RVU, which insurers change every year, is further adjusted according to its Geographic Practice Cost Index, or GPCI, to reflect cost-of-living differences across the country.

My point in describing some of the technical minutiae governing the computation of FFS medical payments is to demonstrate how absurdly complicated and unwieldy this medical payment model has become. Its designers apparently believed that an unending effort to more precisely measure and define medical treatments would allow insurers to evaluate them more accurately. That assumption was wrong. All these refinements have made the computation process more confusing and less efficient. In addition, this overly elaborate coding and valuation system is a blunt instrument that cannot assess the value of every medical service or procedure. For example, how do you assign a dollar value to a conversation about EOL care? I don't believe this can be done using an RVU. This coding system not only fails to measure cognitive care inadequately but also has irreparably damaged the physician-patient relationship.

CODES AND COVID-19

The direct harm that medical codes can cause to patients came to light during the height of the COVID-19 pandemic in 2021. Although most insurers agreed to reimburse treatment for patients diagnosed with coronavirus, that reimbursement had a hitch. The treating physician or the hospital had to use one of the new medical codes assigned to COVID-19 related illnesses. One example of a related illness would be severe acute respiratory syndrome (SARS). If the code assigned by the physician or hospital didn't have this COVID-19 connection, there would be no insurance payment.

As a result, wrote *New York Times* reporter Sarah Kliff, "patients who have tried to take advantage of their insurers' cost waivers . . . are sometimes thwarted by hospitals and providers not meeting the insurers coding requirements for COVID-19 reimbursement. Without the right coding, the patient's normal deductibles and copayments were applied."[1]

The writer noted that a coronavirus patient in Chicago "spent 50 hours trying to get the coding for an MRI scan changed to show it was related to coronavirus. His efforts," wrote Ms. Kliff, "failed to resolve the issue. He is still waiting to see if he will have to pay the full $1,600 charge for the diagnostic procedure."[2]

"I've heard so many stories of people being completely stymied filling out reimbursement forms and trying to get insurance to cover them," Senator Tina Smith (D-Minn.) told Ms. Kliff.[3] Senator Smith is the lead sponsor of a bill to make coronavirus treatment free. "It is almost as if the system is designed to make it hard to get reimbursed."[4] Rather than helping patients during this national health crisis, the medical coding system made a grave situation even more frightening and uncertain.

If a medical provider either mistakenly or purposely lists an incorrect code on billing paperwork, their payment may be denied, they may be charged an astronomical fine, or worse yet, they may be charged with defrauding Medicare, which is a felony that can lead to loss of license and imprisonment.

THE HIGH COST OF COMPLEXITY

Due to the draconian consequences of miscoding, caregivers have been forced to create expensive, time-consuming administrative procedures to ensure that they are complying with the coding requirements. As a result, researchers have found doctors and nurses today spend an inordinate amount of expense and professional time on paperwork and other administrative tasks unrelated to treating their patients. In the *New York Times*, Dr. Danielle Ofri cited a study in which researchers found that the doctors they personally observed for more than four hundred workday hours "spent nearly twice as much time doing administrative work as actually seeing patients: 49 percent of their time versus 27 percent."[5]

After noting that numerous other published studies have documented this same phenomenon, Dr. Ofri concludes, "Medicine has devolved into a busy work-laden field that is slowly ceasing to function. Many of my colleagues believe that we've reached the inflection point at which we can no longer adequately care for our patients."[6]

This fundamental shift in how caregivers use their time has been detrimental to the doctor-patient relationship particularly in treating elderly patients at the end of life. These patients need social support and a relationship with their caregivers, who often are too bogged down in paperwork to give them the time, attention, and critical advice they need to navigate their final years with dignity and comfort. A multitude of studies have shown that having such doctor-patient conversations often improves patient outcomes and raises patient quality of life.[7] Time pressures on primary care practitioners also means they rarely have time to consult with the other medical specialists involved in treating their elderly patients to coordinate their care.

Too often insurers use their excessive documentation requirements to delay payment to providers. The insurer, for example, may not approve the format of the provider's information or the insurer may decide the documentation is incomplete. In an insurance reimbursement environment that resembles the Tower of Babel, each insurer can create its own documentation format and decide what type of information, and how much of it, healthcare providers must submit to them.

Moreover, insurers today demand that caregivers demonstrate in their paperwork that each service they provide is medically necessary. It is more difficult to establish the medical necessity of mental health or addiction counseling or EOL care choices than, say, chemotherapy for a patient with a cancerous tumor, and if something is difficult to measure in the medical insurance world, it is poorly reimbursed. Heart surgery, for example, is easy to measure and thus it is well paid. A primary care visit, by contrast, is difficult to quantify so it is poorly reimbursed. If this devaluation of primary care services continues, millions of elderly patients will miss out on what they need most: the counseling and empathy of their doctor.

Because of insurance companies' inordinate paperwork demands and delay tactics, healthcare providers have come to accept that their requests for reimbursement can take six to eight months or longer to be processed and paid.

Physician David Belk in *The Great American Healthcare Scam* expresses the frustration felt by countless American doctors today when he complains,

> Doctors have very little influence on, or even understanding of, the process by which we are paid. The insurance companies have effectively excluded us from understanding the source of our own incomes. This clearly shows the degree to which health insurance companies have almost complete and unchecked control over the finances of healthcare in this country. If that doesn't worry you, it should.[8]

For an excellent illustration of how destructive this payment model is to the clinical management of care, just look at the management of high blood pressure—one of our nation's greatest health issues. An article titled "Controlling High Pressure: An

Evidenced-Based Blueprint for Change" calls for changing physicians' approach to managing blood pressure.[9] The article's recommendations, at their core, require physicians and a team of caregivers to spend significant time talking with their patients. Additionally, they require delivery system relationships that are aligned and harmonized. In short, they require care coordination not fragmented care. The research documents a critical point: "Dissemination of guidelines without more intensive behavioral change efforts is not useful to facilitate implementation of practice guidelines."[10] Despite all this, these important changes will never see the light of day in FFS reimbursement.

The strategy to implement these changes unrealistically calls for increased collaboration by caregivers. Such a request will fall on deaf ears because the proposals will inevitably be viewed as another unfunded mandate for physicians. No matter how we try and seek cooperation, it will not occur unless we change how physicians are paid. *Physicians cannot afford to spend their time in a way that conflicts with how we pay them.* Unless we change the payment system to support physicians talking with their patients, best practice clinical guidelines will not be adopted.

Congress seems to fundamentally misunderstand the impact of the FFS model's wastefulness and dysfunction. Instead, federal lawmakers have focused on making affordable, government-based, healthcare insurance available to more Americans. That was President Barack Obama's primary goal in creating the Patient Protection and Affordable Care Act of 2010, the most substantive healthcare reform legislation enacted in the United States in nearly half a century. Expanding coverage was also the central component of Medicare for All, a proposal made during the 2020 presidential campaign by Democratic candidate Senator Bernie Sanders. He proposed that the federal government provide healthcare insurance to every U.S. citizen—as is done in virtually every other advanced democracy except ours. However, no recent or proposed reforms have addressed the more critical problem of fixing the expensive and broken FFS model. Legislation in 2021 requiring hospital price transparency is an example of Congress fixing the wrong problem while creating more problems. Hospital pricing is irrational because the payment system is irrational. More transparency and more regulations will not fix that fundamental problem.

CAPPING PHYSICIANS' MEDICARE PAYMENTS FAILED TO FIX MUCH

By the 1990s, Medicare was experiencing an explosion in the cost of physician services under its now decades-old FFS model. Congress's solution was to pass a law placing an annual cap on Medicare payments to physicians. To maintain their existing income levels, some physicians responded by increasing the number of tests and procedures they ordered for their patients.

Eventually the reductions in Medicare payments to physicians were seen by virtually everyone as both ineffective and unfair. Rather than pass comprehensive new legislation to correct the problem, federal lawmakers voted instead to annually override the payment cap. Congress was thereby able to partly appease the doctors, but it has failed miserably in its attempt to contain rising Medicare costs.

Meanwhile knowledgeable observers were discovering other major cracks in the FFS model. According to Shannon Brownlee, author of *Overtreated*, "We spend between one fifth and one third of our healthcare dollars on care that does nothing to improve our health."[11] Ms. Brownlee argues that this wasteful healthcare spending is

> the natural out-growth of our fee-for-service healthcare system. It turns doctors into piecemeal workers who are paid for how much they do, not how well they care for their patients. Doctors and hospitals depend on the volume of work for their income. In addition, they are the gatekeepers who decide when work needs to be done. They also worry about being sued if they do too little. So, they err on the side of overtreatment.[12]

Ms. Brownlee, an award-winning healthcare journalist, is not the first person to notice this problem. We have known for decades in this country that the flaws in the FFS model cause widespread overtreatment, fraudulent Medicare billing by unethical practitioners, and billions of dollars in wasted and unnecessary healthcare spending.

ADDITIONAL REFORM ATTEMPTS

There have been numerous regulatory initiatives to address these concerns by Congress. We have tried capitation, a system of medical reimbursement wherein the insurer pays the provider a set annual fee per covered patient. This approach works well for large, comprehensive healthcare systems such as Kaiser Permanente. The Kaiser model is unique and consists of three distinct groups: medical groups with thousands of physicians; hospitals and outpatient clinics with several hundred facilities; and insurance entities that have millions of enrollees. This level of scale allows capitation to work well for Kaiser, but capitation doesn't work as well for most healthcare providers that lack this scale.

About a decade ago, Congress woke up to the fact that FFS does *not* recognize differences in quality. So for example, a poorly done surgery is paid at the standard insurance reimbursement rate even if many mistakes were made. If an ER physician misdiagnoses a patient—and even if his or her mistake proves fatal—the ER doctor will be paid at the same rate as a colleague in the ER who diagnoses his or her patient correctly. About ten years ago, Medicare and other insurers started to add quality measures to the FFS system. Doctors who could prove they satisfied the insurers' criteria for high-quality care received a slightly higher level of reimbursement. However most physicians found the additional quality-reporting requirements burdensome and the financial rewards for raising the level of patient care modest.

In 2014, Medicare introduced a new program called Accountable Care. It gave participating providers, known as Accountable Care Organizations, or ACOs, a financial incentive to lower the overall costs incurred in treating Medicare patients. ACOs that were able to reduce those costs to a targeted level while maintaining a high quality of care received a percentage of the savings they brought to Medicare as a cash rebate at the end of the year. When I first became aware of this program, Mercy Health, the Cincinnati-based Catholic healthcare ministry for which I served as president and CEO, decided to participate in this Medicare initiative. Theoretically at least, it sounded to me like an everybody wins scenario: Our patients would receive superior care, Medicare would save money, and Mercy Health would get a portion back for every dollar we saved the federal insurer. We were able to enroll 120,000 participating patients. This made us the tenth-largest ACO in the nation.

As it turned out, however, the move did not work out for us—at least not initially. Although we were able to deliver significant savings to Medicare through better care coordination, fewer ER visits, and fewer nursing home days, and though we achieved excellent patient outcomes, participating in the Accountable Care program caused us numerous headaches. Moreover, despite receiving the annual rebate, we ended up losing money. It cost us around $20,000 per doctor per year to satisfy the federal health insurer's elaborate reporting requirements. Perhaps more significant is the reality that physician practices are forced to work under multiple payment models (i.e., Accountable Care, FFS, Medicaid, and Commercial). Each of these different payment models has different economic incentives. These conflicting financial incentives are confusing and frustrating for physician practices to manage.

At the time, I saw Mercy Health's disappointing experience with this new Medicare program as a classic example of how even the most well-intentioned efforts often become entangled in a web of red tape. Eventually however, Mercy became more proficient at meeting the Accountable Care program's elaborate reporting requirements. Today the healthcare system is achieving a modest financial gain by participating in this Medicare reform program while providing excellent care and saving Medicare significant funds. Even so, programs like Accountable Care have done little to change the overall problems in healthcare.

THE MACRA AND MIPS REFORMS

In 2015, just a year after Accountable Care was introduced, Congress enacted another federal measure creating a new FFS framework by attempting to reward healthcare providers for giving better care instead of more care. This law replaced the reimbursement cap discussed above and implemented by Medicare nearly twenty years earlier to control Medicare spending on physician services. However like too many other well-meaning attempts to reform the FFS model, MACRA is needlessly complicated and difficult to implement. Rather than achieving its intended purpose of improving the quality of care, the legislation has added a new layer of complexity to the reimbursement process by creating a multifaceted measurement system known as MIPS (Merit-Based Payment System).

MIPS has *220 different performance measures* organized into four main categories: quality measures, weighted at 45 percent; interoperability measures, weighted at 25 percent; cost measures, weighted at 15 percent; and care delivery improvement measures, also weighted at 15 percent. Each year the patient care provided by eligible professionals (i.e., doctors treating Medicare patients) is assessed by the federal healthcare agency using the MIPS quality criteria described above. Based on their annual MIPS score, the healthcare providers receive either a payment bonus from Medicare, a payment penalty, or no payment adjustment. Doctors performing poorly can face a 9 percent drop in Medicare reimbursements. The most highly rated physicians, by contrast, can see their rate of reimbursement for Medicare patients rise as much as 27 percent. Despite the added financial incentives, however, as with previous measures aimed at improving the quality of healthcare delivery to Medicare patients, MACRA's real-world impact has been negligible.

In a rare bit of good news, on January 1, 2021, Medicare adjusted its physician fee schedule, boosting the reimbursement rates of PCPs by 3.75 percent. These adjustments were budget neutral so the modest pay increases to PCPs reduced payments to specialist practitioners such as cardiologists, orthopedic doctors, and gastroenterologists. Needless to say, the specialists who were set to lose income in 2021 were not happy about these new rate adjustments, and their lobbyists quickly persuaded Congress to moderate the cutbacks with some temporary pandemic stimulus funding.

FFS HAS REDUCED PATIENT ACCESS TO PRIMARY CARE PHYSICIANS

One of the most serious, albeit unintended, problems caused by the FFS model is a dramatic decrease in patient access to PCPs in this country, particularly elderly and indigent patients (I consider family practitioners, internists, palliative-care physicians, and geriatricians PCPs).

The fundamental problem is financial. Reimbursement rates for patients insured by Medicare and Medicaid are lower than those paid by private health insurers. Medicaid rates are substantially lower than both private and Medicare rates. Most physicians are reluctant to care for Medicaid patients because of these extremely low payment levels. This does not make them greedy or heartless. It makes them realistic. Practically speaking, they cannot stay in business if they lose money every time they treat a Medicare or Medicaid patient.

While most physicians do take on Medicare patients, the inadequate payment level for these federal insureds tends to be exacerbated by the difficulties that often are encountered while working with geriatric patients. These patients are more easily confused and thus physicians need to spend more time talking with them and their family members to ensure that their care plan is clearly communicated and carried out. This same point can be made regarding Medicaid patients, who often face additional social problems that require more of the physician's time to sort out.

Each year, millions more Americans become Medicare and Medicaid eligible, adding billions of dollars in new healthcare spending and putting new strains on primary care providers. This problem will only grow worse due to a disturbing, if understandable, trend. Far fewer medical school graduates today are choosing primary care specialties. It's a matter of economics. Primary care is poorly compensated under the FFS model, and few physicians can afford to choose these specialties after an expensive medical education.

The impact of inadequate reimbursement of primary care providers by federal and private insurers combined with a dearth of primary care providers has produced crowded hospital ERs across the country. The ER has become the de facto provider of primary care to millions of poor, elderly, or uninsured Americans and to undocumented immigrants. A recent Commonwealth Fund survey found that "45 percent of lower-income adults reported turning to hospital emergency departments in the past two years (2019 to 2021) for much more costly care that could have been delivered by a primary care provider, had one been available."[13] In addition, an ER visit is a poor substitute for a primary care visit. The ER doctor is not likely to know the patient's health history and often will perform numerous tests to help make a diagnosis. ER physicians also must test patients more comprehensively due to a heightened fear of malpractice claims.

ER visits are particularly disorienting for older patients with multiple health issues. When a self-sufficient older patient visits the ER, often for a minor injury, it can trigger a rapid functional decline. For example, an article in the *AARP Bulletin* by Kenneth Frumkin discusses this post-hospitalization syndrome.[14] The author describes a healthy and active ninety-year-old who had fallen and broke her wrist. She went to the ER and was hospitalized for her wrist injury. This initial visit resulted in the patient's rapid decline. Approximately one out of every five ER visits by people over sixty-five results in multiple hospitalizations even when the initial visit was for a minor injury like a broken wrist.[15] One out of ten of these individuals will die within ninety days of their initial ER visit.[16] Researchers consider the stress of hospitalization itself rather than the nature of the original illness the trigger for the rapid decline. In effect, the older patients' homeostasis is lost during these visits to the ER and the hospital. Easy access to primary care, instead of ER visits, could reduce these risks.

Unsurprisingly, ER visits are far more expensive than primary care visits and contribute significantly to the rising cost of healthcare. One sure way to decrease the volume of ER visits and to provide a higher quality of care to people who now use the ER as a default doctor's office would be to substantially increase the Medicare and Medicaid reimbursement rates to PCPs. However both the federal government and many state governments, which split the costs of Medicaid, have been reluctant to increase these reimbursement levels. While such an action may have some logic, that logic focuses on the belief that we can accurately measure everything. We don't measure the benefits of primary care very well. This obsession with quantitative evidence to justify paying PCPs better prevents us from using common sense to address this issue. The government's faulty measurement analysis tells legislators that increased reimbursement for primary care cannot be justified.

The growth of urgent care centers is another illustration of poor access to primary care. Over the last two decades, urgent care has grown dramatically in response to poor access to primary care. While this new care option does meet a need in the health system, it also contributes to our nation's problem with fragmented care (see chapter 14). The urgent care center generally has no patient history for the patients it sees, and its actions are not integrated well with the rest of the health system. Overall it is cost effective, but it is not care effective. Alternatively, improved access to primary care would be a much better solution.

The current growth in alternative medicine is a further indictment of primary care's failure.

> Alternative medicine appeals to many chronically ill people precisely because it offers what its name suggests: an alternative to a vast, bureaucratic, impersonal medical system that leaves little room for the personal side of illness. . . . A 2016 NIH survey found that Americans were spending $30.2 *billion* a year on alternative and complementary medicine. The desire for care is one reason so many people turn to it. . . . Where conventional medicine focuses on fixing, integrative medicine focuses on healing and prevention. . . . While I had great faith in science, I had begun to see that I stood on the edge of what medicine knew, and that the . . . data-driven, evidence based approach, had run out of things to offer me.[17]

Patients seeking this route exacerbate the problem of fragmented care. These patients feel compelled to leave the system by looking for an alternative, and the ability to integrate the patient's healthcare history is lost. Properly structured, primary care could incorporate many of the caring components of alternative medicine. However, today's reimbursement world makes that accommodation virtually impossible.

These reductions in doctor-patient contact, due in large part to flaws in the FFS model, has led to another disturbing trend. Rather than spend time with their patients trying to better understand their health challenges and more thoughtfully exploring the underlying cause of their pain or anxiety or hypertension, many doctors today simply write a prescription for a drug they believe will address the patient's complaint. In effect, pills have replaced comprehensive conversations between doctors and patients.

FFS HAS HURT THE HEALTH SYSTEM
IN COUNTLESS WAYS

There is no shortage of research to confirm that U.S. healthcare is complex and inefficient and rewards quantity over quality of care. Solving these problems will require abandoning the FFS model and replacing it with a more straightforward physician payment model. The best first step in that reform transition would be changing how we pay PCPs.

So as we've seen, FFS payment produces many negative consequences for the health system. It

- prevents physicians from spending adequate time with their patients. This means physicians no longer get to know their patients and are not easily available to answer patient questions or implement best practices that require time with a patient.
- prevents physicians from talking to one another about their shared patients. That's why today we have an explosion in fragmented care (see chapters 14 and 18).
- adds layers of cost to the health system. As a result, the cost of complying with an insanely complex coding system requires new staff, expensive consultants, and elaborate IT support. The costs and interruptions created by these systems are far more expensive than the alleged efficiency FFS is believed to create.
- enables the insurance concept of medical necessity. This insurance mechanism, in essence, doublechecks a clinician's judgement using prescribed or coded care. My contention is that this approach interferes with the physician-patient relationship while being both unnecessary and costly.
- has created a new fraud and abuse (FA) industry. FA terrifies providers and adds a new layer of unnecessary staffing and consultants that providers now need to hire to protect themselves. These consultants are very costly. FA could be eliminated by a change in the payment system.

The FFS system hurts the physician-patient relationship in fundamental ways. First, FFS uses a measurement system that does not address the real needs of the patient. Second, it rewards caregivers for engaging in all the wrong behaviors. The alleged solution to these two problems is value-based payments, a complex idea that has not yet been fully implemented after decades of effort. Regardless of the approach adopted, however, payment reform needs to be universal by including all insurers and all providers. Partial solutions only create conflicting economic incentives.

The *Harvard Business Review* recently addressed some of these concerns:

> There is widespread agreement that the United States must expand and improve primary care in order achieve better outcomes at a lower cost. . . . For primary care, the conversation with the patient and the longitudinal relationship with the whole-person approach are necessary to achieve results that impact outcomes and costs. Overly concentrating primary care—through policy, payment mechanisms, and infrastructure design—on distinct processes tied to metrics diminishes the powerful role that the patient's relationship with their primary care physician should play in healthcare.[18]

In the next chapter I discuss how we could restructure physician compensation to address all these issues.

13

CHANGING THE PRIMARY CARE PAYMENT MODEL

Change has no constituency.

—Jack Welch, former chairman and CEO of General
Electric Corporation

There are innovations in physician compensation that demonstrate improved patient care, but those innovations have failed to make a meaningful impact on care delivery because they have no scale. Specifically, it is challenging to change physician behavior when physicians need to function under multiple conflicting payment models. Understandably, physicians respond to the dominant model of payment, which for them continues to be FFS. So innovative new payment models have had a negligible impact and do little to change overall behavior. What is needed to make reform effective? A comprehensive payment change is necessary to ensure a better care paradigm. The first step in finding the path forward is to learn from the innovations that have proven successful.

TELEHEALTH

Telehealth is a way of consulting with your physician online in a format similar to a Zoom call. Telehealth has been around for over a decade but at first it was not widely used. Its adoption was limited because of FFS billing practices. The insurance standard of medical necessity did not quickly approve telehealth visits. Moreover it was an uncomfortable and complicated process for physicians and patients to use. Then came COVID-19, and telehealth became a much better treatment option for both patients and physicians. With uncharacteristic responsiveness, health insurers (led by Medicare) quickly decided to reimburse these virtual visits by deeming them medically necessary. Telehealth is a mode of care that is quickly accessible, cost-effective, and efficient for both the patient and the physician. It is particularly convenient for patients. Its use could help address the shortage of PCPs by identifying visits that require a physician's physical presence for determining the best treatment plan. It is particularly effective for mental health visits and urgent care–type visits. It is also a resource to improve access to specialty care in communities that don't have good access to these specialty services. The technology supporting the use of telehealth has also improved, making it more user-friendly for patients and physicians. Similar to how business Zoom calls have changed corporate meetings, telehealth can change how individuals receive healthcare. This technology will never be a complete replacement for person-to-person contact, but it is a valuable and helpful adjunct.

Telehealth may be particularly well suited to improve access to palliative care. Telehealth is one of the most effective ways to connect family members and patients with a palliative-care team. Telehealth can also help patients get answers to their questions about care options more easily than a traditional office visit. Given the absence of palliative care in the outpatient setting, telehealth may be one of the few ways we know of quickly making outpatient palliative care more available.

However, telehealth is now under attack. With the immediate COVID-19 crisis waning, telehealth is again being challenged. Specifically, its status as free of the medical-necessity test is now under question. To add salt to the wound, the fraud and abuse industry has also identified telehealth as a target. Healthcare should embrace, not resist, telehealth. It is a valuable tool to care for patients because it responds to unmet patient needs and enhances physician access.

DIGITAL MEDICINE

Consumers want more control and more immediate feedback on their health status. So digital medicine is on the rise. Sophisticated new electronic devices, such as the Apple Watch, allow us to measure our pulse rate and blood pressure and even count the number of steps we take during an indoor or outdoor walk while calculating the calories we burn. These tools, which do not necessarily require the involvement of a physician, have enhanced our ability to manage and improve our health. They also have engaged patients in managing their own primary care.

One concrete example of how cost-effective digital medicine can be involves my own heart. A few years ago I had a minor stroke. Often it is not possible to know what triggers a stroke. One common cause is an irregular and high heart rate. Today cardiologists use a loop recorder to track a patient's heart rate over time to determine whether irregular heart rates occur. I had a loop recorder implanted in my chest to follow my heart rate and discover whether a heart rate irregularity had triggered the minor stroke. After two years, the loop recorder had found no heart irregularities. In retrospect, it is my opinion that an Apple Watch could have replaced this expensive loop recorder solution. Once the battery in the loop recorder wore out, which took less than two years, I used an Apple Watch instead. I was not going through another expensive procedure to monitor my heart rate. The Apple Watch monitors my heart rate effectively at virtually no expense. Even so, simple technology like the Apple Watch has not yet been embraced by or integrated into the health system.

CONCIERGE MEDICINE

Physicians' dissatisfaction with today's experience in primary care practice has led to a marketplace innovation called "concierge medicine." This is a payment model that allows patients to pay an extra annual fee to improve access to their PCP. This approach uses that additional fee to reduce the number of patients under the care of the concierge physician, thereby improving each patient's access to that physician.

On average, a PCP needs between 2,200 and 2,500 patients to operate an economically viable practice.[1] Given these patient volume requirements, most PCPs do not have an adequate amount of time to get to know and spend time with each patient. The concierge model solves this dilemma by limiting the physician's number of patients to approximately six hundred. This number gives the physician more time to forge a bond with each patient and provide them with better care. To make the economics work, the annual fee the concierge physician charges each patient is usually between $2,000 and $3,000. Using the latter figure, a concierge doctor with six hundred patients would receive an extra $1.8 million per year in revenue over and above what his or her non-concierge patients would pay for an office visit or treatment through insurance.

Many affluent patients gladly pay this additional concierge fee for greater access to their doctor. Surprisingly, these patients also save insurers a tremendous amount of money. The insurance companies benefit because concierge patients, on average, have one-third fewer ER visits and one-third fewer hospitalizations than traditional patients.

The downside of concierge care is that it reduces overall patient access to PCPs because of the drastically reduced size of each concierge doctor's practice (600 patients vs. 2,300 patients). In addition, few patients are in a position to pay the Concierge fee.

DIRECT PRIMARY CARE

There is a more recent variation of concierge medicine known as "direct primary care." In this practice model, the relationship between doctor and patient is similar to that in concierge medicine in that the patient's employer, labor union, or insurer (for example, a Medicare Advantage plan)—pays the PCP a membership fee. This fee covers "extended visits, clinical, lab and consultative services, care coordination, and comprehensive care."[2] Notably, this financial arrangement has led to the formation of large, corporate medical practices.

One significant difference between these two alternative payment models is that direct primary care patients often pay lower or no fees because their fees are being subsidized by their employer or group. Insurers such as Medicare Advantage plans and self-insured employers favor these practice models because they know that making primary care readily available to patients reduces overall healthcare spending per patient. Similarly, physicians prefer these practice models because they are relieved of some FFS billing burdens, which saves on both labor and capital expenses.

Though successful, these variations on FFS primary care only benefit a small segment of the U.S. population. They do not solve the overarching problems caused by the FFS model—namely, expensive overtreatment, mountains of superfluous paperwork, and limited access to PCPs for millions of Americans and particularly those most vulnerable: the poor and frail elderly. Moreover, because concierge medicine is only available to those who can afford it, the payment approach is socially unjust. On the other hand, both concierge medicine and direct primary care show that changing our healthcare payment model is possible and can be done in a way that benefits both the patient and the physician. We need to find a way to accomplish these critically important goals on a larger scale without reducing patient access to primary care.

CHANGING THE PRIMARY CARE PHYSICIAN PAYMENT MODEL

My years as a healthcare system executive taught me that even the most complex, daunting problems can often be solved. One such problem is reimbursement for PCPs. To fix this problem, we should no longer use a coding system to determine these physicians' payments. We should eliminate coding when calculating how insurers pay PCPs. We should also stop the medical-necessity review for primary care services.

This chapter limits its focus to PCPs because they are the healers most likely to be helping patients plan and prepare for EOL care as well as guiding and supporting them and their family members during an EOL crisis.

We need a simple and single payment methodology that allows logic and common sense to determine PCP compensation—not a Byzantine coding system with a thousand moving parts that needlessly complicate and prolong the reimbursement process. Furthermore, we need a payment model that rewards quality of care and not the volume of patients passing through a physician's door or the number of tests or procedures they perform on them. Healthcare insurers should pay PCPs for the services they provide to patients on a reasonable cost basis with some additional features elaborated on below.

Under this revised approach, insurers would reimburse PCPs for the actual cost of providing office care, including nurses, nurse practitioners, IT expenses like electronic records and telehealth, rent, malpractice costs, staff, supplies, and so forth. Physicians would be free to negotiate a reasonable salary within a prescribed range with insurers. This reasonable cost reimbursement payment model has been used before by Medicare to reimburse hospitals but never individual doctors. It could be further refined by making payment enhancements based on standardized measures for quality of care and productivity. A physician who demonstrably provided high-quality care to their patients, measured by positive patient outcomes, could use this information to negotiate a slightly higher salary.

Since most primary care visits involve essential services such as a physical examination, a simple diagnosis, or a sit-down consultation, using an elaborate coding system for payment is irrational. Primary care consumes just 5 percent of the healthcare dollar. Putting these modest costs through a complicated coding and billing process, as happens today under the FFS system, often costs as much as the care itself. The old business adage "Don't use an expensive solution for an inexpensive problem" certainly applies to paying for primary care.

Reasonable cost reimbursement would eliminate the need for coding and most billing for these practices. Additionally it would eliminate Medicare fraud and abuse concerns because overutilization has no financial gain. Because these physicians would be better compensated for patient consultations, PCPs would no longer have a financial incentive to boost their meager Medicare reimbursements by ordering unneeded medical tests or procedures or by quickly referring patients to a specialist to save time. This streamlined payment model would allow them to focus on what they *should* be focusing on: caring for their patients. The time they formerly used to spend on coding and other administrative chores could now be used to see more patients and to spend more time with each of them.

Eliminating coding also would prevent insurance companies from delaying payments and disputing coverage over the issue of medical necessity—actions they have been getting away with for years under our code-driven billing and reimbursement system. Under this revised payment model, *all* primary care visits would be automatically deemed medically necessary by Medicare and all other health insurers. Imagine how much time and paperwork this simple procedural change would save. In addition, primary care patients covered by medical insurance would have no copays or deductibles. The latter reform would economically incentivize patients to go to their primary care doctor first to evaluate their health issues. Then if they chose to go to a specialist or a hospital ER instead, they would face both copays and deductibles. Some insurers have already implemented this change in their policies after discovering that incentivizing covered patients to see their primary care doctor, rather than a specialist, can save them money and improve care.

Replacing the FFS model in primary care with reasonable cost payments would be relatively simple. Over the years the healthcare industry has accumulated extensive data on the cost of providing primary care. That knowledge, coupled with today's sophisticated data management systems, would enable insurers to evaluate reasonable costs accurately.

However, despite this model's efficacy, health insurers would likely oppose it. This is because they would prefer to stick with their highly inefficient, expensive, and increasingly complicated FFS system. Their reluctance to change is driven, in part, by the fact that they have already invested so heavily in the status quo.

HOW WOULD THIS NEW PRIMARY CARE REIMBURSEMENT WORK?

Under this proposal, nothing would change regarding who is paying whom and for what services. Medicare, Medicaid, and private insurers would still compensate physicians based on patient visits. And the reimbursements would be based on the cost of the physician's salary and the physician's office overhead costs. However, the payment processes would be streamlined and simplified. There would be no billing codes to interpret and no going back and forth between the doctor and the insurer regarding what services are or are not medically necessary. There would only be one payment methodology and not a unique payment formula for each insurer. The reimbursement paid for primary care office visits would be based on actual reasonable costs and the physician's negotiated salary within a prescribed range.

150   *Chapter 13*

This cost-reimbursement approach could then use Medi-care's periodic interim payments (PIP) methodology to make routine payments. Under this model, physician practices would reconcile their PIP payments against their cost report (which is based on reasonable actual costs) on an annual basis. Just as hospitals complete a cost report for Medicare, PCPs would fill out a cost report for all insurers documenting the expenses they incurred while treating patients. Each insurer would then pay their share of the cost report based on their percentage of insured patients' visits in the practice. For instance, if Medicare represented 45 percent of the patient visits, Medicare would pay 45 percent of the office expenses and the negotiated salary. These cost reports would require time and effort to complete but no more than a physician normally would spend on an annual tax return.

This increase in primary care compensation would pay for itself. First, insurers would save money by reducing physicians' office overhead costs through this streamlined billing process. Second, insurers would spend far less on expensive ER visits and hospitalizations because patients with enhanced access to their primary-care doctor tend to be healthier.

Under this revised payment model, uninsured patients would be free to negotiate directly with a provider. If an uninsured patient could not afford to pay for treatment, the physician would be free to write off those charges—something physicians used to do more frequently. Today it is illegal for a doctor to forgive a patient's debt unless they can document that the patient is unable to pay. For example, a physician's practice in rural Virginia once accepted fresh fish as payment for primary-care services. This rational payment system is illegal today, and showing such generosity toward a patient can prove very costly. But don't take it from me. Ask Jennifer Thompson, a medical billing consultant.

> Routinely writing off copays will land [medical practitioners] in hot water with [the] OIG (Office of the Inspector General). They are waiting to fine you millions. Practices are paying huge fines for routinely using waivers (charity care) and writing off deductibles. Understanding when and what amounts you are allowed to write off when your provider is out of network or the patient has a financial hardship can be challenging. There are a lot of legal rules that can trip you up, costing you massive penalties and even jail time.[3]

The laws limiting a physician's ability to write off medical bills or accept in-kind payment hurts countless low-income patients. In fact, the leading cause of personal bankruptcy today in the United States is an inability to pay large healthcare bills.

In this reimagined payment system, PCPs would have 600 patients as opposed to the current national average of 2,300. This of course would require more PCPs, but increasing PCP compensation would—in the long run—motivate more doctors to choose primary care as their specialty. In the short term, better financial rewards might even motivate internists who have abandoned primary care to return to it. Overall this model would not only pay PCPs what they're worth, it would also allow them to focus on their patients instead of patient volume and coding.

HOW MUCH SHOULD PRIMARY CARE PHYSICIANS BE PAID?

According to Doctor-Salaries.com, as of January 29, 2021, U.S. PCPs were earning on average $173,035 a year. I believe that figure is closer to $230,000, but in any case, in the interest of both fairness and boosting the number of PCPs, these doctors should be offered an opportunity to negotiate their salary with insurers.[4] Expressly, government programs would establish a negotiated salary range of $300,000–$350,000 while commercial insurers would establish a negotiated salary range of $300,000–$450,000. Although PCPs would not earn as much as surgeons, these salary ranges would give them an income on par with that of most other medical specialists. All physicians spend approximately $400,000 for medical school and give up four years of their lives to become medical doctors. Their salary levels need to help them recover these substantial expenses, most of which are in the form of debt that will follow them throughout their career. Our country needs PCPs—in part to care for tens of millions of aging Baby Boomers—and higher compensation levels will help us respond to that need.

MORE OPTIONS TO IMPROVE
ACCESS TO PRIMARY CARE PHYSICIANS

Another way to increase patient access to PCPs would be to encourage more of them to hire nurse practitioners (NPs) and physicians' assistants (PAs). This effectively would allow them to substantially increase the size of their practice. These added medical professionals would be a fully reimbursable expense on the cost report without coding and billing for these services. These practitioners could see patients with relatively minor complaints such as head colds or routine aches and pains, allowing the doctor to spend his or her time seeing patients with more serious medical issues. Numerous studies have shown that roughly 50 percent of physician office visits do not require a physician's skill level to properly address the needs of the patient.[5] Yet patients always want to see *their* doctor. This is an unrealistic expectation, but it might change once patients saw that their medical needs were being adequately met by NPs or PAs. It's important to note that this would require the schooling, training, and hiring of many more NPs and PAs.

One more strategy to expand physician supply would be to structurally incorporate telehealth in primary care practices.

GETTING INSURERS ON BOARD
WILL REQUIRE LEGISLATION

As with any major reform, implementing this new payment model would have complications. For example, it would prove difficult to get all U.S. health insurers to agree on a standard, reasonable-cost methodology for compensating PCPs. They also would resist being compelled to adopt a single standardized and limited set of quality and productivity measures to be used in conjunction with salary negotiations. Currently health insurers can create their own unique billing structures and quality measures.

Under the new payment model being recommended, all health insurers would need to be legally required to participate. If they were free to opt out—and I suspect many of them would—the reforms wouldn't work.

A NEW PAYMENT MODEL WOULD IMPROVE QUALITY OF CARE

This healthcare payment model would vastly improve the quality of primary care—particularly for patients dealing with EOL issues. (Chapter 14 will explain in detail how this new reimbursement approach would allow primary care practices to become the first resource for patients preparing AHDs or wishing to learn more about their EOL care options.)

In summary, this revised payment model would save both money and time by eliminating the FFS model's superfluous reporting requirements. Most importantly, it would allow PCPs to establish a closer relationship with their patients. These physicians would be financially rewarded for spending time talking with their patients and with other healthcare providers, resulting in better coordination of overall care. Most physicians would like nothing more than to spend time with their patients, but with today's FFS model, they take a major financial hit for doing so.

In sum, this healthcare payment reform would offer the following benefits.

- creation of a single payment model for all primary care visits
- elimination of the medical-necessity standard for all services from a primary care practice, thus allowing those services to be automatically covered by insurance
- reduction of office overhead by eliminating complicated billing and documentation requirements
- elimination of economic incentives for overtreatment by reimbursing physicians for their time rather than for the medical services or treatments they provide. This important change would virtually eliminate fraud and abuse.
- optimized patient access to their PCP
- increased PCP availability by making primary care medicine more personally and financially rewarding for physicians

- increased PCP leadership in educating elderly patients on EOL care choices
- increased PCP coordination of each patient's care with other specialty physicians, reducing fragmented-care problems
- reduction of ER visits and hospitalizations of patients
- promotion of telehealth to increase the number of virtual primary care visits, allowing clinicians to make more productive use of their time
- reduction in the overall number of specialist doctors' visits and hospitalizations

PILOTING THE NEW PAYMENT MODEL

There would be several ways to pilot this new, code-free, reasonable cost–based healthcare reimbursement approach. One would be for a few U.S. states to adopt it as an alternative payment model. Since health insurance is regulated by the states, this makes sense. However, this would only work if all payers in that state agreed to participate. In order to convince physicians to get on board, the states would need to commit to the new experimental payment model for a reasonable number of years. Another option would be to offer this revised payment model to individual health systems or physicians—again, with a firm time commitment to maintain the pilot.

Of course universal implementation would be an even bolder approach. Although this may sound radical to some observers, it has built-in safeguards. For example, limiting the pilot program to PCPs would be a risk-reducing strategy. Starting small with only a small percentage of healthcare costs and physicians would allow medical providers, health insurers, and healthcare policymakers to evaluate the new approach with limited economic risk.

After the first few years, if the pilot payment model were producing the right benefits and savings, the participating healthcare providers and insurers would then implement it on a permanent basis. If on the other hand it was not saving money and improving the quality of life for both patients and their doctors, participants would return to the FFS model.

Again, the FFS model marginalizes the human element of the physician-patient relationship and wastes billions of dollars a year on unnecessary healthcare spending. That said, these reforms have not been tested and may not work. However, considering the deeply flawed status quo, it seems that almost any approach would be better than what we have. And of course, the only way to find out is to try.

I will let President Franklin D. Roosevelt have the last word on this subject given his substantial experience with and powerful approach to complex problems. Upon entering office at the height of the Great Depression, Roosevelt introduced bold measures (some would say radical) to address America's staggering financial crisis. When a reporter asked the president what he would do if his programs didn't work, the president had a simple response: "Take a method and try it. If it fails, admit it frankly, and try another. But by all means, try something."

14

MAKING COMFORT CARE MORE ACCESSIBLE

There are many reasons for the flight away from facing death calmly. One of the most important facts is that dying nowadays is more gruesome in many ways, namely, more lonely, mechanical, and dehumanizing; at times, it is even difficult to determine.

—Elizabeth-Kubler-Ross, MD

Of all the EOL healthcare treatment models, hospice and palliative care are often the most humane. However, many terminally ill patients today do not receive a clear explanation of these comfort care options or they are not made aware of them until it's too late. Considering that Medicare has been covering hospice as an insured benefit since 1982, it is astonishing these services are not more widely utilized today, but it is also explainable.

There are many reasons for the underutilization of hospice and palliative care. First, these two services are disconnected from the traditional healthcare system. Many doctors and insurers do not see these services as medically necessary. Physicians are focused on curing their patients, and insurers only choose to cover medically necessary services. Thus it is unlikely that terminally ill patients will be offered EOL care counseling or comfort care services—or even be told that such counseling and treatments exist. In today's healthcare environment, it takes a proactive patient or physician to offer timely access to either hospice or palliative care. And it will require a fundamental shift in how many Americans perceive these alternate options before more patients embrace them.

According to palliative-care physician Jessica Nutik Zitter, that change in attitude cannot begin until we take the fear out of hospice care. Right now, she asserts, hospice has "a serious marketing problem."[1]

"To lay people," Dr. Zitter explains in *Extreme Measures*, her book on EOL care in America, "[hospice] meant the end of life, no more hope. To physicians, it signaled personal failure—an admission that they couldn't keep the patient alive."[2] On the other hand, Dr. Zitter notes, "once we explained to our patients that the research demonstrated palliative care and hospice care are almost always going to improve the quality of life, most of them were interested."[3]

One major obstacle is that no caregiver is officially in charge of EOL care. Consequently it is unclear who is responsible for guiding patients through this process. Also, neither the patient nor the physician wants to admit the obvious: that the patient is dying and there are no good treatment options left. Further complicating matters is that there are often multiple physicians caring for a single patient, and it is unlikely that one of them will step up and recommend stopping treatment.

In the final analysis, the patient must decide to stop seeking curative care. This heartbreaking decision requires courage, wisdom, and reflection. It also requires an adequate education on the available EOL care options. Yet few patients today are offered support in learning about these EOL care options.

As I've noted, PCPs should become the go-to source for educating patients about their EOL care choices and helping them formalize their intentions in an AHD.

REMOVING THE ELIGIBILITY
BARRIERS TO COMFORT CARE

Appropriate insurance coverage is fundamental to making hospice and palliative care more accessible and allowing people to die naturally at home. Changing the current insurance rules and expanding coverage for palliative and hospice care would significantly improve access to these vital services.

Currently Medicare recipients access hospice through a separate insurance program called the Medicare Hospice Benefit (MHB). For a patient to become eligible for this coverage, an independent physician must certify that the patient has a life expectancy of six months or less. Predicting when a patient will die is difficult. Moreover, these predictions also put the doctors into an untenable position. What doctor would want to say to their patient "I'm sorry to have to tell you this but you will be dead in less than six months"? This somewhat morbid requirement is arguably one of the reasons physicians are reluctant to recommend hospice care.

In another twist, MHB policy also requires prospective hospice patients to give up their doctor and regular Medicare insurance. This policy thinks that standard Medicare coverage is for curing patients and hospice coverage is for easing a dying patient's natural death. You cannot have both curing and caring simultaneously from Medicare.

There is robust evidence to suggest that these Medicare eligibility barriers are misguided. Instead of separating hospice into a distinct, medically unnecessary benefit, Medicare should include it as part of standard insurance coverage. This insurance coverage change would eliminate the beneficiary's need to give up regular Medicare coverage. It would not require a physician to certify that a patient will die within the next six months. Of course there would still be standards for accessing the hospice benefit.

Hospice should be made available to patients with cancer, congestive heart failure, chronic obstructive pulmonary disease (COPD), kidney failure, Alzheimer's, and other potentially terminal illnesses. This approach would integrate hospice into the course of medical treatment so that hospice would no longer be narrowly focused on the last weeks of care. Instead it would become a flexible benefit that is more broadly focused on caring for individuals who require various medical services. This approach would hopefully diminish the death stigma and the marketing problems associated with hospice enrollment noted by Dr. Zitter. It could also lead to earlier palliative and hospice referrals, better quality of care, more prolonged patient survival, and cost savings.

While researching this chapter, I discovered that Medicare has been piloting a similar approach to EOL care on a small scale since January 2016. That is when the federal insurer initiated the Medicare Care Choices Model (MCCM). In this pilot, qualified beneficiaries received both curative care and hospice comfort care services simultaneously.

To qualify, a beneficiary had to be suffering from at least one life-threatening severe illness. In addition, just as with the MHB benefit, the beneficiary's doctor had to certify their life expectancy was six months or less.

According to an evaluation of this still-ongoing pilot program, "MCCM led to a 25 percent decrease in total Medicare expenditures . . . by reducing inpatient care through increased use of MHB for 3,603 Medicare beneficiaries."[4] Both patients and caregivers gave the pilot favorable reviews.

A dozen years earlier in 2004, the insurance company Aetna piloted a similar program offering insurance coverage to critically ill beneficiaries for both curative and comfort care. The Aetna pilot produced similarly positive outcomes of saving money and improving patients' satisfaction with their care.

To me, the evidence emerging from these hybrid hospice programs is a compelling story. Adopting a mixed approach to EOL care by reimbursing both curative and comfort care has been an unqualified success. Patients were happier, and insurance companies not only did the right thing but also saved money in the process. These results strongly suggest that access to palliative and hospice care should be expanded and streamlined. Removing insurance barriers limiting that access would reduce our nation's medical costs and improve patient care.

SIMPLIFY THE PAYMENT METHODOLOGY FOR HOSPICE

Medicare's obsession with coding all services for patients means that this complex medical billing strategy now burdens hospice. Much like primary care services, hospice does not require elaborate coding. Merely paying for these services on a reasonable cost basis, as defined in chapter 13, would make compensation for these services simpler and fairer. Medicare's use of the ICD-10 coding system for hospice has generated the same problems—namely, caregivers spend too much time on documentation to ensure payment and avoid draconian penalties. This elaborate payment structure for hospice care incentivizes the wrong behavior: more time on documentation and less time with the patient.

In addition, as with primary care, there should be no application of the medical-necessity test to hospice services. Anything reasonably necessary to care for a dying patient would be reimbursed without the need for second-guessing clinical judgments. Hospice services are both medically necessary and socially necessary. There is nothing wrong with combining caring services and modest curing services. If it keeps patients out of the ICU, it benefits everyone.

IMPROVING ACCESS TO PALLIATIVE CARE

According to Dr. Diane Meier, a distinguished practitioner of palliative-care medicine in New York City, "Everything important in health care has to do with the relationship [between the physician and the patient] which requires space and time. We ask [patients] what's on their minds, what distresses them the most, what their hopes are, and then we work to move the barriers out of the way."[5]

Dr. Meier believes the importance of comfort care in modern medicine became more evident during the pandemic. When traditional medical practitioners in hospitals around the country ran out of cures for dying COVID–19 patients, she says, they increasingly turned to palliative-care doctors such as herself for help and advice. "While the practice of [curative] medicine is pretty good at the mechanics of treating things that cause tremendous suffering," she told a reporter for the *New York Times Magazine* in March 2021, nonmedical aspects of treating critically ill patients are often placed in the hands of palliative-care teams.[6] "We see that as part of our job," she said. "In the rest of medicine, clinicians *don't*, and people are left to find their way."[7]

Though its value is indisputable, palliative care has been marginalized because it is so poorly reimbursed by healthcare insurance. Insurance views this treatment as not medically necessary. Moreover, it is not easy to find supportive codes for palliative care in the ICD-10 coding system because comfort care is difficult to measure. Creating a new medical specialty to help those facing serious or chronic illnesses and then inadequately funding it is not a rational healthcare policy.

As chapter 13 argues, palliative care should be deemed a form of primary care. In that framework, patients would have access to comfort care services without satisfying medical-necessity requirements. Insurance companies would reimburse that care just like any other aspect of primary care. Under this approach, palliative care could be provided in outpatient as well as inpatient settings so patients could receive this benefit before ending up in the hospital.

One of the great virtues of palliative care is its focus on the needs of both the patient and their family members. Whether a patient receives comfort care at home or in an institutional setting such as a hospital or nursing home, the palliative-care team sits down with the patient's family to answer any questions they might have and update them on the patient's progress and prognosis.

EXPANDING HOMECARE FOR HOSPICE

A foundational hospice concept is putting responsibility in the hands of family members. This is ideal, but in practical terms it is not always possible. For example, not everyone has a family member available to support them. Even when family members are available, they don't always have the luxury of time to do what will be required.

"People believe, and in many cases are led to believe, that hospice care means caregiving" by homecare workers visiting the patient's home, writes palliative-care nurse Sallie Tisdale.[8] "[But] that's not what hospice services do."

When hospice is provided at home, family members must handle day-to-day support tasks such as feeding, bathing, and giving medication to the patient. According to Ms. Tisdale, to receive insurance coverage, the patient's family must "guarantee that a patient will never be left alone."[9]

Arguably Medicare and other insurers could expand homecare services as part of hospice. They could, for example, add up to three hundred hours of homecare support as a lifetime Medicare benefit for enrollees. This might prove costly, but it also could help avoid hospitalizations that would be even more expensive.

We should also consider expanding the scope of practice and training for homecare workers and increasing their wage rates. These changes would attract more people to care for the sick and the elderly at home. There is a growing shortage of homecare workers, and this problem will become even more urgent as America's elderly population continues to explode over the next decade.

Allocating more of our healthcare dollars to homecare services for the frail, elderly, seriously ill, or dying would more than pay for itself by reducing the demand for more expensive hospital treatments.

ADVICE FOR FAMILIES NEEDING TO PLACE A MEMBER IN A NURSING HOME

Nursing homes operate under challenging circumstances. They have modest insurance reimbursements, they function under oppressive regulation, and they are constantly looking for staff to work in challenging situations for fair compensation. Unfortunately, a nursing home is the only option for many individuals.

One of the regulatory issues nursing homes deal with is the public reporting of their death rate. No one wants to go to a nursing home with a high death rate. So the consequences are that nursing homes frequently transfer patients with any potential of dying to the hospital. The nursing homes want their patients to die at the hospital so their own death-rate numbers don't suffer. In many cases, these transfers to the hospital activate the death trap.

If you must use a nursing home, look for one with a hospice component. If this service is available, move from the nursing home and into the hospice unit and avoid the death trap.

ENTRUSTING A LOVED ONE TO HOSPICE

My sister Patricia Ann Connelly spent most of her career helping college students obtain financial aid. In her mid-fifties after years of heavy smoking, she was diagnosed with chronic obstructive pulmonary disease (COPD). COPD is a daunting disease because it gradually takes away your ability to breathe. It took Pat a while to accept her diagnosis and give up smoking, but once she got on board, she was a model patient.

Difficulty breathing was her most significant challenge. When this began happening more frequently, her pulmonologist put her on oxygen twenty-four hours a day. Because canisters of the life-giving gas have now been miniaturized and made portable, Pat could continue many of her normal activities such as grocery shopping and other routine chores.

Predictably the disease progressed, making it more and more difficult for Pat to breathe even with her continuous oxygen feed. Her doctor prescribed steroids to reduce the inflammation in her lungs. Of course steroids have various adverse side effects, so her physician placed limits on her access to steroids. Clinically his concerns were not unwarranted. However, given Pat's limited life expectancy, these concerns about side effects may have been excessive. The pulmonologist was reluctant to renew her prescription without her visiting his office. Though he was trying to protect my sister's welfare, his conservative treatment strategy backfired. While he was on vacation, Pat experienced another breathing crisis. Unable to turn to her doctor for help, she sought relief in the ER of her local hospital.

The ER physicians initially thought Pat's breathing difficulties were heart-related. They admitted her to the hospital and ran an extensive battery of tests on her. No cardiac issues were found. The doctors would have saved themselves a lot of time and trouble and wasted medical expenses if they had listened to Pat when she showed up at the ER seeking help. All she needed was steroids to help her breathe. That is what they finally gave her after two days of expensive and unpleasant diagnostic testing.

On returning home, Pat quipped, "They should replace the death penalty in Wisconsin with a trip to the hospital."

But there was an upside to Pat's tortuous hospital visit. It convinced her that she needed a different approach to her care. I advised her to ask her PCP about obtaining palliative care at home. I suggested palliative care because Pat's mindset was not yet ready for hospice. Her doctor admitted he was unfamiliar with the palliative-care option (this was almost a decade ago) but in time he referred her to a hospice that offered some palliative care.

At this point Pat had realized that only she could decide how she would spend the balance of her days. When the assessment certified her for hospice, she accepted. It helps to bear in mind that her pulmonologist originally suggested she consider a lung transplant, and that neither her pulmonologist nor her PCP ever proactively suggested hospice to her even though her advanced COPD was terminal.

Pat did seriously consider the lung transplant option. However, after we discussed it together candidly, and after I explained to my sister what I knew about this grueling and highly risky treatment course, she decided against it. It is worth noting that a lung transplant would have cost Medicare well over a million dollars while hospice for the remainder of her life was closer to $75,000.

By enrolling in hospice, Pat made a wise and brave decision. Of course Pat was not eager to face death. But like our late mother, my sister was practical, and she was willing to do what she believed needed to be done.

In hindsight it is clear that my sister's timing was most fortunate. Her daughter Christi, an elementary school teacher in Washington, Pennsylvania, was able to spend her two-month summer vacation living with and taking care of Pat. She brought along her ten-year-old son Mitch. If Christi had been unable to do this, our family would have hired home healthcare workers to help look after Pat. Though my brother and I were willing to roll up our sleeves to help care for Pat, neither of us had the luxury of taking a long-term leave from our jobs. In that regard, our family is typical. To make hospice work, more generous insurance benefits are needed since homecare workers often need to be hired to care for an ailing patient at their home.

My sister died five months after enrolling in hospice. She was sixty-five years old. Her courage and determination to seek a different path for her care despite her doctors' reticence allowed her to live out her days the way she wanted. She was able to put her life in order and spend particular time with her daughter and grandson. And there were no more tortuous hospital or ER visits.

Pat's positive experience with comfort care is rare. Most terminally ill patients either do not receive hospice care or enroll too late and thus do not receive the care that could have significantly improved their final months. Most are also not allowed to die where and in the way most of us would choose to die: at home and surrounded by our loved ones.

To make such a natural end available to more Americans, we must remove three significant barriers. First, we need patient education to take the fear out of hospice care. Second, we need to encourage physicians to recommend hospice in a timely manner as a liberating and empowering option for terminally ill patients. Third, we need to remind insurance companies how much money they could save by more generously funding comfort care, including homecare, before a patient's medical condition turns critical. The odds against achieving all three of these goals are not high. It would be equivalent to winning the trifecta in the race for better EOL care. But if any of these three significant barriers were eliminated, it would be a win for U.S. healthcare.

15

NEW FUNDING OPTIONS FOR
END-OF-LIFE CARE

Progress is impossible without change, and those who cannot change their minds cannot change anything.

—George Bernard Shaw

Chapters 13 and 14 asserted that making primary and comfort care
more available to U.S. citizens at the end of life will pay for itself. The
logic behind this position is that these care options are substantially less
expensive than hospital care, so increasing these care benefits pays for itself. But what if those savings don't materialize? What if offering humane
and dignified care to more people raises healthcare spending, which is
already strained to the breaking point? This is an economic possibility
that cannot be ignored. While I intuitively believe these new care options would pay for themselves, I cannot provide measurable evidence
to support my opinion. Therefore I propose implementing the following three financial reforms to fund expanded comfort care benefits. Not
only would these changes fund any increased spending on end-of-life
comfort care, they also could save U.S. taxpayers in excess of $500 bil-
lion every year.

FIRST RECOMMENDATION:
TAX HEALTHCARE BENEFITS LIKE WAGES

There is no rational reason that healthcare benefits should not be taxed
like wages. Healthcare benefits are a component of compensation.
However, numerous studies carried out by the Massachusetts Institute

of Technology and other respected research institutions have shown that not taxing healthcare benefits, which is current U.S. tax policy, encourages overutilization of healthcare.[1] Knowing this, President Obama tried to include a provision for taxing expensive healthcare insurance policies in his sweeping healthcare reform measure, the Patient Protection and Affordable Care Act. Known informally as the Cadillac Tax, this healthcare finance reform was meant to be an important source of revenue to fund the Affordable Care Act, but federal lawmakers deleted it from the proposed legislation before it went into effect. They bowed to pressure brought to bear by a powerful and unlikely coalition: large states such as California and New York in which many residents have expensive healthcare benefits along with anti-tax groups and labor unions.

The late health economist Uwe Reinhardt, a renowned professor of political economy at Princeton University, summed up the issue well:

> Employer-sponsored health insurance receives a generous public subsidy toward their coverage, a generosity that rises with the income of the employee. . . . The sanctity of this public subsidy has long been the third rail of politics. [The value of this subsidy] is estimated to total $250 billion a year—closer to $300 billion if state taxes are included. That subsidy is 2 1/2 to 3 times greater than the entire subsidy given to low-income Americans under Obamacare.[2]

Reinhardt noted that this oft-overlooked but very expensive tax benefit is regressive, meaning it penalizes those with low incomes. If it were eliminated—that is, if employees with a Cadillac level of healthcare insurance had to pay an additional tax for that privilege while those with more modest Ford or Chevrolet plans were not taxed—there would be substantial economic benefits.

The estimated $300 billion in additional income generated by the new tax could be used to help fund Medicare and other government healthcare programs. That was the intent of the Cadillac tax provision. Second, taxing health benefits would incentivize all parties—patients, providers, and healthcare insurers—to pursue value in their healthcare choices; that is, to make choices that are less expensive and that would save them—and ultimately U.S. taxpayers—money.

Today each of these parties is incentivized to spend more, not less, on healthcare. Patients, and especially those whose medical expenses are generously reimbursed by medical insurance, have no incentive to consider cost in making healthcare treatment decisions because there is little or no financial penalty for choosing the most expensive option while healthcare providers are currently paid according to the number and expense of the treatments they provide. The more billable procedures they complete, the more they get paid.

The least likely contributor to overspending on healthcare treatment, one might think, would be private healthcare insurers. Improbable as it may seem, however these insurers actually earn higher profits from the higher-cost healthcare treatments they reimburse. Very little private insurance actually insures healthcare. Rather, most private insurance plans provide employers with an insurance policy that passes through the cost of employee claims and then charges an administrative fee. Under this arrangement, the insurer is paid more for more expensive claims.

To summarize, not taxing healthcare benefits is a policy that is unfair to lower-income individuals. Taxing health benefits, on the other hand, would motivate patients, providers, and insurers to seek cost-effective care options and would generate up to $300 billion a year in additional tax revenue that could be used to help fund healthcare programs such as Medicare. Finally, imposing a Cadillac tax would almost certainly decrease demand for high-cost healthcare treatments, a move that could save hundreds of billions in annual healthcare spending.

SECOND RECOMMENDATION: ELIMINATE ADVERTISING FOR PRESCRIPTION DRUGS

The pharmaceutical industry is a major player in the U.S. healthcare marketplace. It spends billions of dollars each year marketing its products directly to consumers through the advertisements it places in print and online media and broadcast and cable TV. Today the average American television viewer watches *nine* drug ads a day.[3]

Supporters of these ads argue that the drug manufacturers use the ads to inform patients about diseases and potential treatments; to encourage people to seek medical advice; to help cure illness; and to provide revenue for drug research.

Opponents of so-called direct-to-consumer advertising argue that drug ads misinform patients, stimulate an artificial demand for drugs, medicalize normal conditions like wrinkles, waste medical appointment time, and, most significantly, have led to an overuse of prescription drugs.

I believe the evidence demonstrates that the problems caused by this flood of pharmaceutical ads far outweigh the benefits. The pharmaceutical industry's goal is not to help the consumer, as its apologists claim, but rather to sell more drugs by appealing to consumers who are desperately seeking a cure for life-threatening ailments such as cancer, congestive heart failure, and diabetes. It is important to note that this magical-cure marketing campaign has been going on for years. In a 2006 study of 221 cancer patients published in the medical journal the *Oncologist*, the doctors who were treating these patients reported that

> 94 percent of patients had made a request for an advertised drug, and 40 percent [of these oncologists] said they experienced one to five requests per week. Alarmingly, 74 percent of the physicians said patients asked for an inappropriate drug, which 43 percent [of these doctors] said they sometimes felt pressured to prescribe.[4]

It would be difficult to find a more glaring example of drug manufacturers injecting themselves directly into the patient-doctor relationship in a way that can be financially wasteful or clinically harmful (if an inappropriate drug were prescribed) or both.

The American Medical Association (AMA) found this situation so disturbing it called for a ban on all direct-to-consumer prescription drug advertisements in 2018. However, even one of the country's most powerful medical lobbies failed to reverse this trend that had begun more than two decades earlier. The drug advertising boom began in 1997 when the U.S. Food and Drug Administration relaxed guidelines relating to direct-to-consumer advertising on broadcast media. Since then the growth in spending on prescription drugs in this country has exploded. Pharmaceutical spending has gone from roughly 7 percent of total healthcare spending in the early 1990s to over 17 percent in 2015, and by 2019, Americans were spending more than half a trillion dollars on prescription drugs annually.[5] A research report published by the University of Pennsylvania's Wharton Business School tied the huge increases in pharmaceutical spending directly to the pharmaceutical industry's aggressive ad campaigns. Its authors noted the "substantial effects of advertising on drug utilization. We estimate that a 10 percent increase in advertising exposure increased the number of prescriptions by about 5 percent annually."[6]

Artificially stimulating demand for prescription drugs through advertising has proven costly. According to Alpert, Sood, and Lakdawalla, a 10 percent increase in spending on drugs by U.S. consumers and insurers results in an additional $55 billion annually in drug spending.[7] Eliminating direct-to-consumer drug ads would recoup a substantial portion of these misspent funds. An alternative means for limiting the damage caused by aggressive drug advertising would be to impose a substantial new tax on advertisers, forcing them, in effect, to help pay for the increased demand for prescription drugs that they are creating or, even better, discouraging them from running the ads at all.

Perhaps the most powerful illustration of how detrimental drug advertising is to our nation's healthcare system comes from the books *Empire of Pain* by Patrick Radden Keefe and *Dopesick* by Beth Macy. These books powerfully demonstrate the lengths to which pharmaceutical companies go to promote drugs like Valium and OxyContin and to artificially stimulate demand for their products.[8]

THIRD RECOMMENDATION: LIMIT MEDICARE REIMBURSEMENTS FOR GEOGRAPHIC VARIATIONS IN EXPENSES

While taxing benefits for commercial health insurance for non-retirees will generate significant government revenue, this action will not impact Medicare recipients. However there is a strategy to encourage Medicare enrollees to live in low-cost Medicare states. This strategy could save billions.

The Social Security Administration (SSA) pays enrollees a standard monthly retirement stipend based on their work time contributions. Medicare, which also serves retirees, handles their benefits differently because its benefit varies in cost depending on where the recipient lives. Medicare reimburses hospitals and other healthcare providers based on the cost-of-living differential for their geographic region. In certain metropolitan statistical areas (MSAs), which are officially determined by the U.S. Office of Management and Budget, medical providers receive higher Medicare reimbursements ostensibly due to the higher cost of healthcare labor in that region of the country. Medicare determines these regional healthcare labor costs using its Medicare Wage Index, or MWI. This is yet another clunky and arbitrary Rube Goldberg invention that was put into service by Medicare more than thirty years ago.

Like so many well-meaning efforts by federal healthcare officials, using the MWI to calculate healthcare labor costs is unnecessarily complicated and inefficient. During the implementation of this new regulation, Medicare officials decided that healthcare represented a unique labor market and thus the cost of healthcare labor had to be tracked by geography for reimbursement purposes. This task was done through the elaborate data collection process Medicare uses to gather financial information through hospital cost reports. In my view, Medicare did not have to use this complex data collection approach to adjust its reimbursement based on regional labor costs. Medicare and health lobbyists insist on keeping this complex, time-consuming reimbursement model in place and have refused to use the easily available cost-of-labor data gathered each year by the U.S. Bureau of Labor Statistics (BLS), which has adjusted for regional cost variations for decades. The BLS data would be far less expensive to use and arguably more accurate than the Medicare's own, essentially redundant, data. But like the ICD-10 coding system that dominates the U.S. healthcare payment system, the federal government is willing to spend vast sums of money to make these complicated, and perhaps unnecessary, calculations.

More importantly, Medicare uses the cost of healthcare labor data it collects in a way that favors healthcare providers in certain regions of the country while shortchanging providers in other regions. According to one research article, average Medicare spending per enrollee in 2014 was $10,936[9] but there was significant variation among states ranging from a high of $12,614 spent per Medicare enrollee living in New Jersey to a low of $8,238 spent for an enrollee living in Montana.[10] In other words, healthcare providers in New Jersey were paid 53 percent, or $4,376, more by Medicare than healthcare providers in Montana for the exact same service.

Distributing federal healthcare funds based on regional labor costs is wasteful and unnecessary and should be stopped. Making this change would save the federal government billions of dollars in wasteful spending. If it is a good policy, why doesn't the SSA use it?

One way to reduce these geographic payment variations would be to eliminate the use of the MWI altogether. We should standardize Medicare payments to healthcare providers just as the SSA standardizes its payments to enrollees living in all parts of the United States. The SSA does not make cost of living adjustments based on where an enrollee lives. Why should Medicare do things differently? As a result of its skewed regional reimbursement policy, this federal insurer effectively makes healthcare providers in poorer states subsidize their counterparts in richer states by giving the former significantly lower Medicare reimbursements.

A less radical reform option would be to limit the amount of regional variation allowed in Medicare reimbursements. For example, the variation might be limited to 10 percent above and 10 percent below the average service payment for labor costs. This approach would be consistent and less complicated to implement.

CHANGING THE STATUS QUO IS NEVER EASY

The financial reforms proposed in this chapter—taxing health benefits, eliminating direct-to-consumer pharmaceutical ads, and making Medicare reimbursements uniform across geographical regions— are long overdue. They are simple, commonsense reforms, and none of them would be difficult to implement. However, these policy actions require trade-offs.

It may take a political visionary to step onto the national stage before we can begin to resolve the problems in our healthcare finance system that urgently need to be addressed. For perspective, it is important to keep in mind that even in the unlikely event that all three of these recommended reforms were adopted, this would not save anyone in this country from falling into the death trap of default curative care. However, these reforms are worth fighting for because they would make comfort care easier to fund and thus available to many more people. In my view, this would be an excellent trade-off and a good way to start changing the way we die.

16

REINSTITUTING THE ROLE OF CARE COORDINATION AND CREATING A HOME

A large part of the task is helping people negotiate over-whelming anxiety—anxiety about suffering, anxiety about loved ones, anxiety about finances [which requires time with a patient]. There are many worries and real terrors. No one conversation can address them all.

—Dr. Susan Block, palliative-care physician at Harvard
Medical School

Patients seldom have the opportunity for in-depth conversations with their physician. The primary reason is physician compensation. A second contributor is hyper-specialization in healthcare. While this specialization has led to tremendous advances, there is a downside: the fragmentation of patient care. This fragmentation falls most heavily on the elderly, who face many chronic illnesses with diverse medications and multiple physicians. These patients in particular need time for conversations with their physician. The concept of patient-centered healthcare was developed as a response to this dilemma. Patient-centered care is more of a theory than a reality, however. The way physicians currently are economically forced to operate keeps them far away from the holistic intent of patient-centered care.

Caring for elderly patients requires more extensive conversations yet no single specialty has the time to handle this critical task. Historically, primary care was responsible for care coordination. A retired geriatrician and internist who's a good friend of mine shared that he used to tell his patients that his job was to keep them from seeing other physicians. Why did he have this approach with his patients? Because he knew that once his patient was referred to another physician, he would likely lose oversight of their care. Today PCPs no longer seek to keep their patients. Rather, it is more likely they will refer patients to someone else due to hyper-specialization and economic pressures.

When I started in healthcare over forty years ago, there were fewer than twenty specialties. I distinctly remember when they first recognized emergency medicine as a specialty. Today there are literally hundreds of specialties. If you combine this growth in the number of specialties with the fact that physicians are not reimbursed for talking to one another, you get today's poor coordination of care—especially for the elderly who need it most.

A PATIENT STORY ILLUSTRATING CARE FRAGMENTATION

Marjorie was a grandmother with a fifteen-year history of Type 2 diabetes. Type 2 diabetes is the most common form of diabetes, a condition in which chronic high levels of sugar can lead to disorders in the circulatory, nervous, and immune systems. This patient also had elevated blood pressure and recurrent episodes of major depression. Marjorie had a body mass index of 37 (she was obese) and had struggled with her weight since youth. She made an appointment with her PCP for progressive fatigue and depression. At the appointment, tests showed her sugar level was too high and her blood pressure was too high, and the patient health questionnaire she had filled out suggested major depression despite her medication for depression. Her PCP decided to postpone adjusting her diabetes and blood pressure medicines until her depression was under control.

Marjorie was referred to a mental health center to review and update her depression treatment. She saw a psychiatrist who had received no information about Marjorie before seeing her. Marjorie arrived for her appointment with extremely high blood pressure and complaints of headaches and fatigue. The psychiatrist was alarmed by these symptoms and sent her immediately to the ER. At the ER, another physician told Marjorie that her blood pressure medicine was inadequate and that she needed new and more powerful medications. She received prescriptions for two new medications to combat her high blood pressure, but it wasn't clear to her how the new prescriptions related to her old prescription, so she took both sets of blood pressure medications.

One week later, Marjorie fainted while rising from the toilet. She was transported by ambulance to the nearest hospital where she was found to have neurological deficits and was admitted to the hospital with a possible stroke. With adjustments in her medications, her blood pressure stabilized, and the neurological deficits cleared, she was sent home with another appointment at the mental health center for her worsening depression.

Once home Marjorie became increasingly depressed, forgetful, and dysfunctional. She didn't have the energy to go to the mental health center and increasingly became less diligent in taking her medications. Three weeks later Marjorie's daughter found her apparently paralyzed in bed. Marjorie was immediately admitted to the hospital with a serious stroke.

Marjorie's PCP was dismayed to hear about this course of events from the daughter. He was unaware of any of the events that had followed her last visit with him. Marjorie's daughter was stunned and angered by his ignorance.

This sequence of events exemplifies fragmented care. Such fragmentation occurs more frequently than we realize. Physician specialties are not communicating or working together. If Marjorie's care had been better coordinated, her stroke might have been avoided. This lack of care coordination is a long-neglected issue. Clarity on how physicians should relate to one another is not one of our advances in medicine. When it comes to care coordination, we need to re-establish primary care's leadership role and make communication among physicians a core value. Under the payment model proposed in this book, primary care practices would be paid to lead such care coordination. However, specialists will also need to welcome this relationship with primary care.

Matthew J. Press, MD, writes, "As a general internist, I often serve as the quarterback for my patients' care—helping them navigate the system, advocate on their behalf, and coordinate their evaluation and treatment."[1] This is how primary care should operate, but for all the reasons outlined in this book, it doesn't.

Dr. Press goes on to describe a patient he identifies as Mr. K. Mr. K was seventy years old and a long-standing patient of Dr. Press's practice.

He'd only had a few minor medical problems when one day he came to Dr. Press with new symptoms. Mr. K had pain in the area below his ribs and above his pelvis and fever. Such pain, if it persists, might be kidney stones, a urinary tract infection, or more seriously, cancer. A subsequent CT scan revealed a kidney stone and a two-inch mass in Mr. K's liver. An MRI confirmed that he probably had bile duct cancer, or cholangiocarcinoma.

Over the next eighty days, eleven clinicians became involved in his care. Mr. K had five procedures and eleven office visits with these other clinicians. During this time Dr. Press, the PCP, had forty communications with other clinicians, Mr. K, and Mr. K's family. While Mr. K's care was superb, there were several instances when Dr. Press's intervention was crucial during the course of all these procedures and treatments.

Dr. Press discusses lessons learned. He specifically suggests that if we wish to provide patients with high quality and safe care in today's specialized and complex healthcare system, then we need better care coordination.[2] Dr. Press further stresses the importance of teamwork and relationships. An experienced nurse navigator could handle many of these coordination components, but certain communications, such as clinical conversations, are best carried out physician to physician.

How was Dr. Press able to achieve excellent care coordination? His stature as an academic teacher-researcher helped especially since his patient load was only one-tenth the typical PCP's patient load. Dr. Press's unique care model resulted in better patient care, and this model is feasible for all clinicians if the policy changes recommended in this book are implemented.

At the core of my recommendations is recognizing that PCPs need to be fairly compensated for the time required to adequately handle care coordination—as chapters 12 and 13 suggest. Furthermore, the other specialties caring for shared patients need to be receptive to primary care coordination. Involving patients in their own care is another strategy to better coordinate care, and that involvement requires patient conversations. In elderhood, this means creating a home for the patient where they can start learning about what to expect as they age and begin planning for their EOL care choices.

ADVANCED CARE PLANNING:
ANOTHER INCOMPLETE APPROACH
TO END-OF-LIFE CARE

Advanced care planning (ACP) focuses on identifying each patient's EOL treatment preferences using a multidisciplinary team approach. This planning aims to identify the patient's preferences before a health crisis and document them in a care plan. Ideally ACP involves both patient and family. The care team works with the family to develop a care plan that reflects the patient's wishes. In addition, the plan should reduce moral distress for family members designed as surrogate health decision makers. An ACP seeks to spell out the patient's wishes and ensure they are carried out.

One progressive health system in Pennsylvania, WellSpan Health, adopted a system-wide approach to implementing ACP. The WellSpan Health system has eight hospitals and 170 outpatient locations. Their initiative was thoughtful and included dedicating clinical staff to support it. They also completed a trial approach to this initiative before adopting it system wide. Part of the initiative included using one particular type of AHD known as the "five wishes." The team also developed educational information for patients on various EOL issues.

The WellSpan System provided this ACP service to over twenty thousand individual patients from 2016 to 2020, finding that "patients with ACP accrued significantly lower costs compared with those without ACPs. Patients admitted to the ICU with ACP had inpatient costs 24.5 percent lower than those without ACP. Furthermore, even amongst patients not admitted to the ICU, those with ACP had inpatient costs 24.5 percent lower than those without ACP."[3]

This evidence is compelling and illustrates the power of regular and formalized conversations and education about EOL care. The evidence suggests that better informed patients and families receive superior care at a substantially lower cost to society. However, the current economic structure of FFS payments makes broad-based implementation of ACP unsustainable. In the unusual case of WellSpan, WellSpan agreed to underwrite the costs needed to support this initiative. This impressive success was an aberration because few systems are financially able to make such a commitment.

Another perspective on ACP is offered by Joan M. Teno, MD, who makes a compelling case for the importance of customized conversations with patients to address the "psychologically complex process of improving decision-making at the end of life."[4]

While she sees value in the ACP tool, she believes multiple tools and plans are needed to effectively help patients with these decisions.

> Our moral obligation as physicians is to help dying persons and their families make important healthcare decisions consistent with their values and to make treatment plans that can accomplish those goals. . . . Simply stated, it is to move on from [a] simplistic single focused [solution] . . . toward multifaceted interventions[5]

Physicians need the freedom to spend dedicated time with their patients to discuss EOL care. When meeting with their patients, physicians should be free to access various tools to meet the unique needs of each patient. This approach to EOL care does not lend itself to standardized billing codes. Physicians should embrace multiple tools—from ACP to videos to other team members attuned to the psychological and social needs of the patient—to address EOL care. Perhaps most importantly they need to be empowered with the economic resources to provide these services.

CREATING A HOME FOR EOL CARE CONVERSATIONS

As we've seen, EOL planning is one of the most neglected elements in the U.S. healthcare system. In part this neglect occurs because no one is clearly in charge of carrying out this responsibility. EOL care planning needs a leader and a home. In my opinion, the PCP's office is the most logical home for these EOL conversations. Indeed, one of my key recommendations is that we formally expand the role of primary care to include care coordination. One critical element of this care coordination would include educating patients on what to expect as they progress through elderhood. Meaningful EOL care requires multiple conversations. Accordingly, a patient's EOL plan and preferences should become a routine topic of conversation with his or her primary care team, including PCPs and qualified nurses. Finally, the patient's AHD should be put in their electronic medical record so that it is easily accessible by patients and caregivers.

The first step begins with helping patients understand that they need to assume responsibility for creating their own EOL care plan. The ideal place to start these conversations is during a PCP office visit. Again, the patient needs to make the important decisions surrounding EOL care, but they can make better choices by being informed about their various care options. It is far better to learn about these options before a crisis situation arises because during that crisis, such decisions will be doubly difficult to face. Therefore, preparing an AHD *before* a crisis and based on *informed* choices is a key recommendation in this book.

Patients may need a nudge to help them assume this responsibility. My proposed nudge is direct: Medicare should require all beneficiaries to have an AHD and a HCPA before getting Medicare insurance coverage. While this may seem draconian, and one might argue that this is an unreasonable infringement on an individual's freedom, there is a counterargument—namely, that Medicare benefits come with patient responsibilities. As the Lancet Commission suggests, we all need to cultivate our own death literacy.

It is also important to stress that knowledgeably completing these documents will have tremendous benefits. These documents are a gift to the families who may need to make critical decisions on behalf of the patient, and they will allow caregivers the opportunity to better understand their patient's preferences. As such, the benefits of this requirement far outweigh their burden.

When it comes to AHDs, shifting from a legalistic focus to an educational one would help patients with their planning. There are many educationally friendly versions of these documents referenced in this book such as the Fitzgerald sisters' compassion protocol (chapter 8) or the five wishes model discussed above. Completing these documents with clinical guidance is highly desirable. We should be sending patients to a physician's office for this support and not to a lawyer or a website.

Each hospital should have a palliative-care team. And if hospitalized patients do not have an AHD, the hospital's palliative-care team should be responsible for assisting them in completing one. However, we also need to offer more clarity on the palliative-care team's role and authority. Hospitalized patients are typically under the oversight of an admitting physician, but due to specialization and economics, there is usually confusion as to which physician should be in charge of taking the lead with patients on EOL choices. This makes for additional confusion between the admitting physician and the palliative-care team.

Unless the admitting physician requests a palliative-care consultation, this team will not see the patient, and for many of the reasons cited in this book, physicians are not prone to seek such a consultation. This lack of coordination needs to be addressed. Patients deserve better access to palliative care. Dr. David Weissman proposed eighteen years ago mandatory consultations for patients near death. This recommendation never went very far. I tend to avoid mandatory solutions because a single mandate doesn't work in all situations. However, we need to find a way to be more proactive with palliative-care consultations. My suggestion is that all specialties actively work on this issue in order to avoid a mandate.

One immediate, structural change that may be worth making would be a mandatory consult—in effect, a trigger whenever a Medicare patient is considering any of the following treatments: a transplant, a ventilator, a feeding tube, entering an experimental clinical trial, or kidney dialysis. Part of this triggering process would include a formal review of the patient's AHD with a palliative-care team.

Preparing primary care practices for these added responsibilities will require new education. Physicians are not trained in medical school or residency to handle these crucial conversations surrounding EOL care. Such training should be required—particularly for each PCP's continuing education. In addition, nurse practitioners should be given the opportunity to gain expertise in this area with an EOL care conversation certification. Given the current shortage of PCPs and their time constraints, making this delegation to nurse practitioners would be sensible.

It would also be helpful if patients understood that getting more healthcare as they age may not always be desirable. Food offers a helpful analogy here. Most of us have a desire for more food (I know I do). We also know that more food isn't always good for us. In old age we may desire additional treatment because of our physical and mental decline. Yet just like more food, additional treatment may not be a good idea. We need to gain an appreciation for this reality sooner rather than later. Although physicians typically find themselves answering the question

"What are my treatment options?" the patient should actually be asking "Will this treatment make my life better or worse?" The difference in perspective between these two questions is critical to EOL care. Dr. Atul Gwande offers insight on this point:

> People have concerns besides simply prolonging their lives. Surveys of families with terminal illness find that their top priorities include, in addition to avoiding suffering, being with family, having the touch of others, being mentally aware, and not becoming a burden to others. Our system of technological medical care has utterly failed to meet these needs, and the cost of this failure is measured in far more than dollars. The hard question we face, then, is not how we can afford this system's expense. It is how we can build a healthcare system that will actually help dying patients achieve what's most important to them at the end of their lives.[6]

So how do we best educate individuals on these issues? Another tool to use is videos. Dr. Angelo E. Volandes of Harvard Medical School has done extensive research demonstrating that patients better understand their EOL care choices when those choices are explained using videos. More specifically, patients were much more willing to move from curative care to comfort care once they understood, after watching a video, what curative care really looks and feels like.[7] But patients don't have direct access to these videos because the videos must be prescribed by an attending physician, and physicians in turn may not be aware of these videos or they may not see them as part of their curing mission.

One may wonder why patients can't access these videos on their own (i.e., without going through a physician). Fear of malpractice is the primary reason. The physician making the videos believes he would be potentially liable for the decisions or acts of a patient who watches one of the videos without the direct guidance of their physician. This risk is eliminated by requiring that the videos come from the patient's attending physician, but it is the patient who ultimately pays the price. The tremendous success of the Gundersen Health System, which has used such videos for decades, is another example of how effective videos are in helping people understand their EOL options. Videos also save valuable clinician time and use non-technical language that patients can understand. Overall, videos need to be offered to more patients. Creating a designated home for EOL care would help make that happen.

And here's another recommendation. We should offer patients an economic incentive to learn about EOL care through videos. Part B Medicare recipients, on average, pay out of pocket to Medicare about $100 per month for their insurance coverage. This is a lot of money for a retired person on a fixed income. My recommendation is to make approved videos on EOL—for example, "Understanding Your AHD"; "Understanding Palliative Care"; "Understanding Dementia"; and "Understanding Hospice"—more available. Upon viewing an approved video, each beneficiary would be given one $100 credit against their Part B Medicare premium. There would be a maximum number of credits—say five per person. This economic incentive would increase individuals' interest in learning about EOL care. My premise is that educated Medicare patients consume less in EOL care, and the savings in care would cancel out the cost of these credits.

Fragmented care and the lack of a home for EOL planning make it difficult to meet the health challenges of the elderly. The first step in solving these problems includes designating a physician to coordinate patient care and providing physicians with the resources needed to carry out these responsibilities. The second step is to create a home for EOL conversations so patients can learn what to expect in their final days. Taken together, these steps will greatly improve EOL care.

17

ACCEPTING LIFE'S LIMITS

Old age is the only disease where you don't want the cure

—Jedediah Leland in *Citizen Kane* (1941)

Americans don't like limits. And we love our independence. But no matter how hard we try, life is limited. It's just like finances. We cannot always afford what we want, but we still want it (just look at our nation's debt levels). The consequences of not accepting limitations, however, will become especially challenging in healthcare over the next decade.

Interestingly, there is one area in healthcare where we have demonstrated an ability to accept limits: organ transplants. We have accepted that there is a limited number of organs, and we have established a disciplined process of ranking patients who are eligible for them. Remember Gerald, the alcoholic mentioned earlier in this book? He was not eligible for a transplant.

As a society, we put limits on distributing organs. This wasn't the only way to arrange things; we could have taken alternative approaches. For instance, we could have sold organs to the highest bidder. Or we could have allowed individuals to sell their own organs, which would have expanded the supply of organs. These approaches to transplants would have commodified organ distribution.

Ultimately our society rejected the commodification of human organs on moral grounds. Instead we created an independent organization of expert clinicians to oversee the allocation of human organs. That organization is the United Network for Organ Sharing (UNOS)—a private, nonprofit organization that supervises the nation's organ transplant system. In other words, we accept the fact that there are limits, and we ration organs by giving them to the individuals who will benefit most.

Yet when it comes to costly new medical treatments, we have not adopted this logical approach. In terms of new medical technology, the cost of not accepting limits will increase dramatically in the next decade. One illustration of this is kidney dialysis. This advance in treatment became generally available in the mid-1970s when Medicare made it a covered service regardless of the patient's age. Since that time the number of patients receiving dialysis has grown from 10,000 per year to more than 500,000 per year, and kidney dialysis now consumes an amazing 6 percent of *all* healthcare spending or $300 billion dollars annually.[1] Dialysis is a treatment for end-stage kidney disease. This treatment requires the patient to go to a dialysis center for four hours a day three to four times per week. The vast majority of these patients die within one year of going on dialysis. This is a classic example of not accepting limits. This illness is called "end stage" for a reason. Yet technology and financial resources allow patients to postpone their inevitable end.

Our immediate future is full of new, expensive technologies like kidney dialysis. Some of the most significant advances will be in stem cell therapy. Today it is possible to treat and cure sickle cell anemia with stem cells—at a cost of $1 million per person, and we have close to 300,000 people with sickle cell anemia in America. Alzheimer's drugs and other stem cell therapy treatments, including new cancer drugs, are being developed that could cost a similar amount.

We should consider getting ahead of these rapidly expanding and expensive care options. We could start by limiting the use of advanced medical technology in the same way that we ration organs for transplants. And I hesitate to use the word "ration" because the word alone provokes a negative reaction in U.S. healthcare. Using this word virtually shuts down any discussion of more balanced approaches to distributing our limited healthcare resources. Why is rationing in healthcare viewed negatively? The alleged reason is that we don't want to put a price on saving a person's life. But one could argue we already ration healthcare. We ration healthcare through our payment system. The classic examples of this rationing are mental health and primary care. We pay poorly for these services and therefore they are in short supply. We pay much more generously for surgery and admission to an ICU, so these expensive services are in abundant supply.

Another rationing example is Medicaid insurance: a wide number of healthcare providers do not accept Medicaid because it pays so poorly. As a result, Medicaid recipients have their care rationed because their access to many healthcare resources is limited. That is why Medicaid recipients use an ER as their PCP. It has always bothered me that different illnesses have significantly different profit margins. Why do different illnesses have different profit margins? Because that is how our payment system operates. This difference in profit margin is a form of rationing we seldom discuss in health policy. Rationing our care based on those who would most benefit from that care seems a much fairer way of rationing than using payment levels to limit access to various types of care.

I recommend limiting costly, new treatments to those who will benefit the most from them. Accordingly, expensive care options like stem cell therapy, kidney dialysis, transplants, ICU admission, and costly drugs for cancer or Alzheimer's should be rationed like organ transplants.

A critical question one might ask is who decides which patients will be eligible for these advanced and expensive services. Few Americans would trust the government to make such personal decisions. But the bigger question is what decision-making process do we wish to use to allocate these limited resources? Before we determine who decides, we need to know the decision-making criteria they'll be using. Today we rely on a payment system and insurance companies to determine the fate of one's access to care. These entities tend to use criteria that are beneficial for them and not criteria that are beneficial for the patient and society. My recommendation is that we change the decision-making criteria *and* change who decides. This approach is not without flaws. There will be flaws in whatever approach we choose to use. However, we need to keep in mind that the real question is not what the perfect decision model is but rather what the best available decision model is. This new approach will not be without controversy, and it will require trade-offs.

This rationing approach to distributing these limited resources would have a disproportionate impact on the elderly. It would limit the elderly's access to these services because the value and success of these treatments for the elderly would be limited. Admittedly this is a radical position, but it is one other advanced nations have accepted for years.

In Britain twenty-two years ago, a quasi-autonomous, nongovernmental organization known as the National Institute for Health and Care Excellence (NICE) was established to develop clinical guidelines for the National Health Service (NHS). Over its history, NICE has gained worldwide respect for its work. There are several unique aspects to their work. First, they integrate evidence-based medicine *and* economic evidence. Their guidelines require completing "a cost effectiveness analysis that takes into consideration cumulative costs and healthcare effects over the time."[2]

In the United States we separate financial implications from clinical care recommendations. We have the National Institute of Health (NIH) along with the specialty medical societies that are responsible for developing evidence-based medical treatment criteria, but these criteria exclude any economic considerations. Additionally, we have an entity known as MedPAC, which is appointed by Congress and is charged with assessing the economic impact of coverage and payment issues for Medicare. MedPAC's charge does not allow it to integrate clinical and economic issues. Efforts to combine these perspectives and implement integrated care solutions as England does are entirely absent in the U.S. healthcare system.

Another unique aspect of NICE is that it integrates medical and social services by viewing them as one continuous benefit. In the United States we separate medical services from social services because medical services are covered by insurance and both services are paid for by different entities. This practice keeps the U.S. healthcare system from effectively integrating social services and medical services. Consequently U.S. healthcare invented the concept of medical necessity to separate medical issues from social issues. Health insurance will only pay for medically necessary treatment, which is why insurers frequently invoke the concept of medical necessity to deny insurance coverage. That is also one of the reasons why hospice and homecare are not effectively integrated with healthcare delivery. But the reality is that medical care and social services are intimately related. Separating them creates a nightmare for patients and is poor public policy.

The acronym "NICE" explicitly acknowledges Britain's commitment to integrate curing and caring as a single benefit. My recommendation is that we would better manage our limited economic resources by following England's example. We need to get over the idea that clinical criteria and economic criteria need to be separated. Specifically, we need to integrate them when we are allocating health resources. Creating an independent organization similar to NICE to guide national health policy would be the best way to do this. This organization would be designed to be free of political or government influence and committed to using the best scientific and economic resources available to decide how medical resources will be provided to patients. This new entity would not be perfect—it would have flaws. After all, donated organs are not always distributed with perfect fairness. However, integrating clinical care and economic consequences will improve our healthcare decisions overall.

American healthcare has avoided integrating economics and clinical efficacy. Yet it is increasingly apparent that the current system is not working. Instead we focus on solutions unlikely to succeed. One current example of this is our focus on healthcare underinvestment in community health.[3] This topic's popularity is based on the obvious observation that social determinants of health have a tremendous impact on health and healthcare costs. So healthcare systems are being encouraged to invest more in social services like housing, food pantries, prevention screenings, and workforce development, the logic being that these social services promote community health.

Yet at the same time we have a payment system that essentially ignores these social determinants of health. Despite a major push in the United States to promote healthcare systems that address the social determinants of health, little progress has been made. Just as the movements promoting palliative care and gerontology lost steam, so too will the movement for social determinants of health. Why? Because these movements ignore economics. Unless we pay for services that we know will save money, we will not get those services. It is a fundamental economic principle.

Instead of the NIH and medical societies developing clinical evidence guidelines while MedPAC develops economic analyses of Medicare spending independently, these activities should be integrated into one independent organization. This new, independent organization would embrace the fact that clinical care and economic realities need to be integrated. Yes, this integration would limit access to care for some individuals, but it would also optimize care for the nation overall. Furthermore, it would be an opportunity to reduce futile care and better manage our limited resources. We already ration healthcare—we just do it ineffectively.

One modest but nonetheless promising illustration of how and why this type of health policy is needed is the Choosing Wisely initiative of the American Board of Internal Medicine. This project was created to encourage a conversation about the overuse of medicine in our country. It is intended to change our culture of medicine to more proactively reduce unnecessary procedures and lower healthcare costs. One example, to illustrate how it works, is the project's recommendation that DEXA bone scans not be used on women under age sixty-five to screen for osteoporosis.

Yet this initiative has had only a very modest impact on actual practices because it is a stand-alone effort that is not integrated into our payment practices. We need a collective, nationwide effort to build real momentum around the need to integrate clinical and economic factors in health policy.

Such initiatives have little likelihood of advancing without general public support. That's why I'm arguing it is in our society's best interests to accept limits on healthcare availability. The economic consequences of ignoring this reality will soon become apparent to all of us otherwise. The clinical consequences of denying this reality will be harmful if we continue promoting futile and unnecessary healthcare. The real question is whether we want to face these realities head on or rather ignore them and so let disaster sneak up and take us by surprise.

18

THE IMPORTANCE OF
ACCEPTING TRADE-OFFS

There are no solutions. There are only trade-offs.

—Thomas Sowell

Thomas Sowell, is, among other things, a University of Chicago–trained economist, author of dozens of books, and a scholar at Stanford's Hoover Institute. For the purposes of this chapter, however, his quotation about trade-offs offers a powerful perspective. As Sowell says, society's greatest challenges require trade-offs. This means that even the best solutions require sacrifice. There is no free lunch.

This book explores trade-offs aimed at improving healthcare and lowering healthcare costs. In particular, this book focuses on the elderly population's special healthcare needs. Of course, making those meaningful trade-offs will require sacrifice and courage.

- What should we change? How about giving up unrealistic expectations about what medical care can accomplish near the end of life? Or how about embracing death in our elderhood?
- What do we hope to gain? The opportunity to die at home with our family around us rather than isolated in an ICU bed and attached to machines.

Decisions about trade-offs are personal and should be guided by individual values. Indeed, coming to terms with these realities requires wisdom. Accordingly, it's worth considering the wisdom of Etty Hillesum. She once observed,

By "coming to terms with life" I mean . . . looking death in the eye and accepting it . . . accepting destruction as part of life and no longer wasting my energy on the fear of death. . . . . It sounds paradoxical: by excluding death from our life we cannot live a full life, and by admitting death into our life we enlarge and enrich our [life].[1]

Etty died at Auschwitz at the age of twenty-nine because she sacrificed herself in order to save another prisoner, one with a young family, from going to the gas chamber. Hopefully her courage and wisdom in facing death will inspire us to face hard choices in old age.

Our political dialogue today rarely asks us to accept trade-offs. When faced with a complex problem, our government usually avoids any unpopular solution. No one gets elected by forcing the public to face hard realities. Our society, in general, seems increasingly unwilling to accept trade-offs. Why is this the case? Honestly there are numerous reasons, but the point is that our society doesn't embrace trade-offs.

Healthcare, in particular, tends to avoid economic trade-offs when making clinical decisions. Healthcare has a narrow focus—namely, the health of an individual. A recent article published in the *New England Journal of Medicine* acknowledges the flaw of this narrow focus. It suggests that healthcare needs to integrate economics with the trade-offs required for public policy.

> Economics is the study of trade-offs that individuals, institutions, and countries face when making decisions under resource and time constraints. Although public health practitioners and researchers understandably focus primarily on improving health, economists view health as one, albeit an important, component of what people may value. This insight is a key aspect of economics utility for informing public health policy. . . . Understanding how . . . trade-offs inform optimal allocation of scarce societal resources will be critical to improving population health, particularly in marginalized populations. . . . A key contribution of economics to public health is the elucidation of complex trade-offs . . . which include non-monetary costs and benefits that are often ignored by policymakers. Economic models can help health policymakers craft more equitable policies.[2]

Trying to use expensive technology to cure individuals of old age instead of supporting their social support needs with palliative care, home healthcare, and hospice is a poor public policy trade-off.

Let's look more thoughtfully at some trade-offs in EOL care. Remember Mary from the introduction, the ninety-two-year-old who followed her doctor's advice to have a procedure with a complicated name that was much like a colonoscopy. Why did she have this procedure? First, she was afraid she might have cancer. Second, the gastroenterologist recommended this course of treatment to help alleviate Mary's fear.

Yes, the procedure confirmed Mary didn't have cancer, however, there were trade-offs. First, the procedure was an unpleasant experience and made her feel pretty miserable for almost a week afterward. Second, there was a less invasive method available of confirming she didn't have cancer. That less invasive option was to change her medications and see if her bleeding stopped. But even if she had cancer, at age ninety-two there wouldn't be any chance of treating it. Changing her pain medication and waiting to see if the bleeding went away would have been the better choice—especially since the outcome was the same. Finally, this procedure was so expensive, financially and personally, that Mary decided afterward the benefits were not worth the expense.

Let me briefly give one more example. This case involves an eighty-two-year-old patient named Betsy. She'd had numerous chronic illnesses, including cardiac disease and diabetes, and her health was failing rather dramatically, but her doctors recommended open heart surgery to alleviate the worst of her symptoms and extend her life. As it turned out, the procedure itself was successful, but Betsy died two months later having never really recovered from the trauma of her surgery.

Why was this procedure carried out? Because Betsy and her family knew she was dying, and they wanted to do everything possible to save her. Were alternative care options presented to her and her family? Did her surgical team provide a blunt description of what life after surgery might be like for Betsy? No. The focus was only on finding the best treatment option to extend Betsy's life. The focus was not on the nature of that life and the impact of the surgery on Betsy and her family.

Needless to say, if Betsy and her family had been able to spend meaningful time before this crisis with clinicians talking about other options like hospice, this painful scenario might have been avoided and hundreds of thousands of dollars would have been saved as well.

Facing life choices like these is difficult but the reality of dying cannot be avoided. However, if you embrace these challenges instead of trying to defeat them, you'll find solace in the fact that a longer life is not always a better life.

Aging forces us to face such issues. In some circumstances, aggressive medical treatment is the best course of action. In other circumstances, letting nature take its course is the best answer. While making those choices is more of an art than a science, the purpose of this book has been to help each of us find a better balance between the two. We can't have it all, and we will need to accept trade-offs. Moreover, we would likely be better off with a bit more wisdom and a little less clinical science when making these choices.

Perhaps the most fundamental trade-off in healthcare will be how to pay for it. Society's increasing demand for Medicare, Medicaid, and Social Security will make such hard choices inevitable. Under today's model, the federal government will not be able to adequately fund these vital safety-net programs much longer. Change is inevitable, and facing these issues head on is better than trying to avoid them. To cite Thomas Sowell again, "People who refuse to face the reality of hard choices are forever coming up with some clever third way—often leading to worse disasters than the hard choices."[3] Clever third ways, like massive deficit spending, only pass our problems on to future generations—with compound interest.

One way to improve our approach to aging is to imagine how we wish to face the end of life. Do we really want to live longer? Or might we aspire instead to focus on a more meaningful life? A fortunate few will have both while many won't have either. Nevertheless, everyone faces difficult decisions about healthcare in their old age.

This book has introduced some controversial ideas—ideas like taxing health benefits; requiring an AHD in order to receive Medicare; limiting differences in Medicare payments driven by geographic variation; changing our FFS billing system; or putting limits on personal autonomy. While these proposals would come with a clear cost, they would better—in the long run—than the status quo. "Clever third choices" are often disastrous.

Economist Uwe Reinhardt believed that healthcare is a social good, and he was gravely concerned with the future impact of the cost of U.S. healthcare.

Over the past four decades, the growth of health spending has exceeded the growth of GDP on average by two and a half percentage points. [This trend] . . . will simply continue to chew up more and more of the American economy, at great expense to America's other, competing national needs, such as education, infrastructure, the environment, national defense, R&D, and so on.[4]

Here Reinhardt defines the fundamental trade-off for society in terms of aging and healthcare. Today's healthcare system is narrowly focused on conquering disease and extending life. But what about how that approach will impact future generations?

Our culture's strong sense of individual autonomy has seemingly displaced our sense of the common good. This book has tried to find trade-offs that are good for both the individual and society. Unbridled individual autonomy in healthcare is one reason why we have a healthcare system designed to try to keep us alive at all costs and in virtually all circumstances. Our sense of personal entitlement to care, our legal system, and our assumption that economic and clinical decisions should be separate, all contribute to this problem.

Initiating steps to override all these forces is difficult. Fundamentally we need to look at ourselves and our values to make *our* choices. A new attitude toward aging will be needed if we are to reform the healthcare system.

We also need to acknowledge there are many valid reasons for our healthcare system as it is. For one, life is valuable. The idea that a human life is priceless is the premise behind saving life at all costs. The real question then is "What is life?" What exactly are we saving? Spending time reflecting on what life really means to us is not just a philosophical necessity, it is a very practical one.

Advances in technology have blurred the line between life and death. Our system errs on the side of keeping our body parts functioning, but are we *alive*? Most physicians and our entire healthcare system assume the vast majority of patients want to do everything possible to prolong life as long as they can. Modern medicine can extend our body's function, but it cannot prevent our inevitable death.

When the end draws near, it is usually preceded by an acute escalation of medical intervention. One-third of elderly Americans undergo a surgical procedure in the last year of life, one-fifth within the last month of life. Given that these procedures are performed so close to death, it's reasonable to ask whether these procedures offered the patient any meaningful benefit.

Near the end we don't often consider that more medical treatment may be futile. Rather, we hope that one more procedure may save us from the end. Not much thought goes into understanding the nature of the existence we are trying to extend.

Michel de Montaigne, a sixteenth-century French philosopher, spent significant time reflecting on life and death. He died at the age of fifty-nine from an infected tonsil—something easily cured today by modern medicine. Did Montaigne in the end feel cheated for not having a longer life? No, instead he embraced death philosophically, equipped with wisdom: "If you have lived one day, you have lived them all. One day is equal to all days. There is no other light, no other night. This sun, this moon, these stars, the way they are arranged, all of these are the very same your ancestors enjoyed and will entertain your grandchildren."[5]

Montaigne helps us focus on the life we have been given and not on the longer life we may desire. Moreover, our choices in facing death should not be guided by science alone—we need to embrace our own values and listen to our feelings and intuition when making these decisions. We need to reframe our thinking about how we seek medical care as we age and incorporate this wisdom.

Comfort care offers us an improved opportunity to weigh these choices more carefully outside a crisis. Yet these consultations are seldom available in primary care practices. Making palliative care and hospice more easily accessible to aging patients would allow them the opportunity to make more informed choices about comfort care. Our healthcare system, however, does not make it easy. It is designed to offer frail elderly patients options like transplants, kidney dialysis, and open heart surgery and not to educate them about comfort care. Making it easy for patients to learn about hospice and palliative care as an alternative to high-tech medicine is possible.

It is the high-tech options, which the U.S. healthcare system promotes, that cost millions of dollars. The comfort care options of palliative care and hospice cost much less, yet they are not easily accessible. This is a trade-off our country's health system doesn't balance very well. Accordingly, this book offers concrete options for restoring the balance.

Another important trade-off is a personal one. Will we choose to learn about EOL care and plan accordingly? Or will we rather avoid planning for elderhood, leaving the difficult choices to our families or the health-care system? Thinking about our mortality and accepting responsibility for articulating our own EOL care plan is as difficult as it is important.

Our society has certainly adopted a proactive stance in preparing for birth and so we educate ourselves when we're preparing to raise a child—Dr. Spock's famous book *Baby and Childcare* comes to mind. And just as preparing for parenting requires effort and education, so does preparing for elderhood. There are many great books on this topic, but one in particular stands out: *A Beginner's Guide to the End*, by B. J. Miller, MD, which is the equivalent of Dr. Spock's book but for elderhood. This book offers practical advice for living life and facing death while Dr. Miller's YouTube channel "Mettle Health" offers educational advice on numerous elderhood issues. All in all, this channel is an ideal comple-ment to the book because it shows us what to expect in elderhood. Another recommended educational resource is Dr. L. S. Dugdale's *The Lost Art of Dying*, which offers practical clinical advice grounded in experience and wisdom.

Another critical aspect to accepting personal responsibility for elderhood preparation relates to our personal aspirations vis-à-vis longevity. While we don't control when we die, we do control how we live. At some point, one might decide that preventative healthcare no longer makes sense. Rather than focusing on preventing and diag-nosing each new health issue, perhaps there comes a time when we are free to let go of those concerns and obligations.

While taking pills and getting check-ups can help (up to a point), there will come a time when it is better to let nature take its course, when high-tech medicine is no longer a choice. This kind of mindset, of course, is one that takes trade-offs into account. We give up the security of trying to treat or know everything that could go wrong with our health in exchange for freeing ourselves to focus on enjoying the time we have left and accept what life gives us without aggressive medical intervention.

THE IMPORTANCE OF WISDOM

The trade-offs offered in this book will not be for everyone. Nevertheless, what is essential is that all of us understand how and why our healthcare system promotes the healthcare it does. Understanding this reality will allow us to be informed about the choices we make. That said, scientific logic and evidence seem to have displaced wisdom as our primary criteria for making decisions. That is a shame, because oftentimes the most sound decisions in life are based on wisdom and philosophical contemplation, not clinical calculations. While the scientific method has unquestionably done wonders for the world, it is not always the best guide to EOL decisions.

In his book *The Unbroken Thread*, Sohrab Ahmari argues that we live in an "age of chaos" that could benefit from a restoration of "the wisdom tradition."[6] Ahmari's book offers a thoughtful plea for humanizing limits and challenging our propensity for modern certainty. He also suggests that unlimited progress has a false allure that cannot satisfy the soul.

For centuries the world's great philosophers and religious traditions have taught that real happiness comes from pursuing virtue and accepting limits. The postmodernism of today's world seems to have unshackled us from these stubborn traditions. We are free to choose the way of life *we* think optimal (or the easiest). One might argue that this approach to living, for all its freedom and independence, is marked by personal isolation and unhappiness. This freedom can be used to avoid trade-offs.

Alexander Solzhenitsyn conveyed a similar message to the Harvard graduating class of 1978 about the implications of unfettered freedom by challenging Western civilization's approach to freedom.

> Every citizen has been granted the desired freedom and material goods in such quantity and of such quality as to guarantee in theory the achievement of happiness. . . . In the process, however, one psychological detail has been overlooked: the constant desire to have still more things and still a better life and the struggle to attain them . . . imprint worry and even depression. . . . Active and tense competition fills all human thoughts without opening a way to free spiritual development.[7]

Solzhenitsyn concludes by criticizing our conception of death. "If humanism were right in declaring that man is only born to be happy, he would not be born to die. Since his body is doomed to die, his task evidently must be of a more spiritual nature."[8]

Solzhenitsyn articulates some of the more important trade-offs we face in life. Perhaps more significantly, he offers an incisive perspective on why we avoid difficult trade-offs. We use our freedom to avoid hard choices. Perhaps the best we can hope for is to use wisdom in making hard choices—choices like preparing ourselves for the end of life and not pursuing our desire to live forever. Doing so would answer Solzhenitsyn's call for us to do our duty on life's journey even when that journey requires us to accept difficult trade-offs.

19

CONCLUDING OBSERVATIONS

> The ability to shape the future sits with us all. The commission believes that profound, rather than incremental, change is needed to transform how we relate to death, and how we die.
>
> —"Report of the *Lancet* Commission on the Value of Death"

I n most cases, death is a gradual process. The process will involve significant interaction with the healthcare system. During this process, difficult decisions will be faced by all involved. This book is about helping individuals, families, and clinicians prepare for those difficult decisions. The first step in the preparation process is to take personal ownership of how you wish to use healthcare in your elderhood. You can become educated and make your own choices, or you can allow the healthcare system to make those choices for you. This book is the beginning of your death literacy education.

This book is also about transforming the health system and the death systems in this country. The proposed transformations are not incremental—they are profound. The recommended changes impact our cultural attitude toward death and our health delivery system. For example, what is our cultural approach toward death? The *Lancet* Commission defines society's death system as follows:

> Death systems are how death and dying are understood, regulated, and managed. These systems implicitly or explicitly determine where people die, how people dying and their families should behave, how bodies are disposed of, how people mourn, and what death means

for that culture or community. Systems are shaped by social, cultural, religious, economic, and political contexts and evolve over time.[1]

So what are today's expectations in our death system? Perhaps one of our most significant cultural expectations is that we want to live as long as possible. This expectation surfaces in families that expect parents to try to live as long as possible and in clinicians seeking to always cure the patient. This attitude illustrates itself in numerous organizations that promote living to be over one hundred. It isn't easy for any of us to accept death. Combine these expectations with our natural fear of death, and you get a health system designed to keep us alive at all costs. Is that what we really should want as a society?

There is an ancient story about someone who tried to live forever, the epic tale of Gilgamesh, the King of Mesopotamia. The story begins with the death of Gilgamesh's best friend, which triggers fears about his own mortality. Consequently, Gilgamesh sets out on a quest for everlasting life. He thinks that as a king he'll find a way to overcome death. While Gilgamesh ultimately fails to live forever, he learns much in the process.

During his journey, Gilgamesh learns about the cycles of life. The annual cycle of spring, summer, fall, and winter becomes a metaphor for childhood, youth, adulthood, and elderhood. Like the changing of seasons and the passing of time, Gilgamesh comes to know life is temporary. So we age, the seasons change, we experience life differently, and our spirits mature. As Gilgamesh learns, the winter of life is a time for accepting detachment from life. This understanding then leads to less dependence on the material world and a greater focus on meaning. In other words, old age is more about *understanding* your life than *extending* it.

While it is difficult to accept death as an inevitability, it is possible for us to do so individually and as a society.

An excellent first step to accepting death is learning what to expect from our healthcare system in old age. This education will help you understand how the U.S. healthcare system views death. This system's narrow clinical mindset and clinical approach to death dominates most people's final days. While this clinical mindset is well intentioned, too often it results in overly aggressive, unpleasant, and expensive treatment. A wise and prepared person can avoid this outcome.

Those who are not prepared often die in institutions—isolated, uncomfortable, and alone—instead of at home surrounded by loved ones. Unsurprisingly, surveys show that most people would prefer to die at home with their family. While dying at home is an option, it takes preparation and effort.

With that in mind, this book takes a holistic approach to EOL care to help you learn how to die at home. It offers a two-pronged approach to reforming care in the United States by looking at the U.S. health system and death system. The first prong is learning how to accept personal responsibility for better managing your EOL care choices. The second prong is reforming U.S. healthcare to offer each of us better access to compassionate care and better understanding of our care choices. Making better use of comfort care options like palliative care, hospice, and home healthcare is at the core of these reform recommendations. Crucially these recommendations can drastically improve the dying process and at the same time dramatically reduce healthcare spending. Each of these recommendations has been discussed in detail in this book, and you'll find them summarized in the appendix.

FRAGMENTED HEALTHCARE IS A COMPELLING PROBLEM CALLING FOR REFORM

This book argues that the FFS payment system, along with hyper-specialization, has created a serious problem: fragmented healthcare. For older patients, fragmented healthcare is particularly dangerous because they and their families can be overwhelmed by the complexity of health-care and not well informed about their options. Such an environment is not conducive to making informed choices. Moreover, even younger, well-educated patients can be frustrated by this environment. Frag-mented care makes it difficult to make good choices.

In chapter 16, I discussed fragmented care's impact on the elderly and on patients with chronic illness. One could argue that old age is a chronic illness. Frankly, most doctors don't like dealing with chroni-cally ill patients. In chronic illness, the patient doesn't have a problem that can be solved. Rather, these patients need physical and psycho-logical support to help them *manage* their disease. Doctors don't like to *manage* problems; they prefer to *fix* them. Medical education emphasizes solutions. The FFS billing system is focused on precise diagnosis and solutions. "According to a *British Medical Journal* study of doctor-patient relationships in chronic illness, the treatment of chronic illness conflicts so fundamentally with these expectations that it tends to be neglected."[2]

These issues have had a profound impact on EOL care. Our health system's economic incentives have further encouraged fragmented healthcare. Let me illustrate these consequences with a story about the impact of chronic fatigue syndrome on a patient. Every year thousands of Americans catch a virus and never really recover. They suffer headaches, brain fog, chills, fever, limb pain, poor sleep, fatigue, and other symptoms as well. Some have described their symptoms as a living death.

Illnesses like chronic fatigue syndrome are difficult to diagnose and tough to treat. Importantly though, these illnesses are in many ways similar to the health problems associated with aging. In both cases, treatment options aren't always clear cut, and finding evidence to support needed treatments is further impeded by the FFS coding system, which requires proof before authorizing payment.

It may take numerous visits and conversations with a physician before finding the best course of treatment—or accepting there may not be one. In fact, patients are often bounced around from specialist to specialist because no single physician is coordinating their care. Why does this occur? Arguably the coding and billing system is cause. The system incentivizes this behavior by not compensating physicians for time spent with patients. If a physician cannot immediately diagnose the patient or find an appropriate billing code to justify his or her time, they typically need to end the visit. As a result, when physicians can't quickly determine a code for treatment, they tend to refer that patient to another specialist. This practice of passing the buck is not only confusing and frustrating for patients; it is poor care and expensive. The elderly especially are passed from specialist to specialist with no understanding of their care plan.

In his memoir *The Deep Places*, Ross Douthat, a *New York Times* columnist, offers a powerful description of how the health system responded to his chronic condition. A few years ago Mr. Douthat began suffering chronic fatigue symptoms. In his memoir, he documents his journey through the healthcare system—a journey that is both sad and absurd.[3] It is also a journey similar to that many older patients with chronic illnesses make. After much trial and error, he eventually discovers—albeit with little assistance from the medical establishment or insurers—that he has Lyme disease.

As this book has shown, our healthcare system, while well intentioned, is rigid, bureaucratic, and often thoughtless. In Douthat's case, when doctors could not explain his symptoms, their response was to blame the victim. Indeed, physicians repeatedly told Douthat that his symptoms were all in his head and that his physical symptoms were actually a mental health issue.

Douthat's story is relevant to EOL care because it chronicles the challenges of chronic illness—and old age is the ultimate chronic illness. As one book reviewer put it, "Chronic conditions tend to share some commonalities . . . physical pain, distress of soul, and social degradation, all at the same time."[4]

Our healthcare billing model does not handle chronic illness well. Accordingly, physicians don't handle it well either. Our billing codes are dependent on established medical evidence and standardization. This approach to care is not responsive to ambiguous pain, mental illness, care coordination, addiction, or social degradation, much less "distress of the soul." These health issues are very real for the sufferers, but they don't lend themselves to easy quantification and standardization. Many chronic conditions, such as the ailments of old age, are fundamentally unmeasurable. A quotation attributed to Albert Einstein comes to mind: "Not everything that can be counted counts, and not everything that counts can be counted." Sinclair Lewis offers us similar wisdom when he observes that our society has "outsized faith in measurement."[5]

While our healthcare system has attempted to address some of these concerns, its success has been nominal at best. For example, the specialties of geriatric medicine and palliative care were initiated to address some of these interpersonal concerns. Yet these specialties are seldom used or available today. Similarly we have a shortage of PCPs because they are under-recognized and under-paid. Furthermore, homecare and hospice are labeled "medically unnecessary" and therefore are under-utilized. However all these services have two crucial characteristics in common: they are about caring for the patient, and they are not about curing the patient.

These observations bring us back to Douthat's book, which discusses the difficulties of chronic illness and our healthcare system's poor response to these difficulties. Modern medicine has trouble diagnosing atypical health issues because, by definition, they do not fit a predetermined diagnostic narrative. For Douthat, Lyme disease was one of those atypical cases. He notes,

> The incentive structures forged by the CDC were a fascinating case study in how bureaucracy shapes science as much as the other way around, how without conscious decision, let alone conspiracy, scientific research can end up pushed again and again down the same well-worn tracks. The narrow diagnostic criteria became the benchmark not just for doctors treating [and billing for] patients but for researchers when they applied for public grants, so Lyme research increasingly focused on only the most certain diagnoses and left all ambiguous cases and all false negatives alone. This approach ratified the establishment's confidence in their own rules of evidence.[6]

In short, our healthcare system doesn't like to deal with illnesses it cannot quantify or doesn't understand. Mental illness, aging, and many chronic illnesses are not well understood. Their symptoms can be ambiguous and hard to measure so they are not easy to treat or study. As a result, these illnesses are often overlooked by the medical, research, and insurance establishments.

Douthat's story connects to EOL care in a number of ways. First, a solely scientific approach to caring for the elderly is incomplete at best. Chronic illness and old age cannot be fixed. They need to be managed with support systems like those anticipated by comfort care. We have difficulty accepting this reality both as individuals and as a society. Instead of focusing on *curing* ourselves in old age, we should focus on *caring* for ourselves. More to the point, caring for the elderly shouldn't be viewed as medically unnecessary. There is strong evidence to suggest that caring would create better patient care and cost less money. Of course modern medicine should use its tremendous resources to treat and extend life, and in many circumstances the results are wonderful— but not always. In old age, the decision to stop treatment is not wrong. It is a personal choice and not a scientific calculation.

Second, incentives determine outcomes. Financial, clinical, legal, and insurance incentives all influence how a health system operates. Today all these incentives drive patients and caregivers to use high-tech medicine rather than simply caring for the individual. This approach is more expensive and results in poor care for the elderly. Overall these incentives serve as a major barrier to dying at home.

Third, Douthat's story is an exemplary account of how destructive fragmented care can be for patients and their families. Of course, fragmented care is an acute problem for the elderly.

This book has offered concrete recommendations on how we can change healthcare incentives, improve EOL care, and create significant savings for our nation. However, implementing these changes will require taking action, accepting trade-offs, and gaining more appreciation for ambiguity, for accepting the reality that not everything a patient needs should be subject to tests of measurement and standardization.

The relevance of appreciating the value of ambiguity in healthcare is well articulated by Meagan O'Rourke: "Thinking about disease as a complex individualized consequence of genes and infections and stress and our immune system means living with uncertainty instead of diagnostic clarity."[7] Healthcare billing and coding are based on diagnostic clarity. Structuring physician compensation to rely almost exclusively on standardized and quantifiable measures destroys the physician-patient relationship.

O'Rourke goes on to observe, "American culture—and American medicine within it—largely strives to downplay the fact that we know so little about illness. A doctor friend told me that in medical school, he was explicitly taught never to say 'I don't know' to a patient. Uncertainty was thought to open the door to lawsuits."[8]

Reforming U.S. healthcare will require all of us to accept two realities: (1) not everything should or can be measured; and (2) we don't know the answer to many questions about our health or otherwise.

A long life is a gift. However, these additional years can come at a price. Often those extra years mean a higher likelihood of encounters with the health system, which can be arduous.

As we've seen, our healthcare system has a rigid directive to keep us alive at *any cost*. While medical technology can and will try to keep us alive as long as possible, mere existence may be worse than death.

We must remember that maximum treatment is an option, not an obligation. In fact, in our waning years, avoiding complicated treatment may be advisable. How each of us deals with age, dying, and death is a personal matter, and so this book offers an approach to preparing for those eventualities.

> Death is for us not merely a fact—something that happens to us. It is an object of reflection. We may not think about it constantly, but the thought of death is never far away, and the ability to think about it is always with us.[9]

How we face our immortality is a spiritual or ethical reflection and not a clinical one. We as a society and as individuals need to re-balance how we approach dying.

APPENDIX

Recommendations for Improving End-of-Life Care

The American medical system is broken. When you look at the rate of medical error—it's now the third leading cause of death in the U.S.—the overmedication, creation of addiction, the quick-fix mentality, not funding the poor, quotas to admit from ERs, needless operations, the monetization of illness vs health, the monetization of side effects, a peer review system run by journals paid for by Big Pharma, the destruction of the health of doctors and nurses themselves by administrators, who demand they rush through 10 minute patient visits, when an hour or more is required, and which means that in order to be "successful," doctors must overlook complexity rather than search for it.

—Norman Doidge, MD[1]

Our [nation's poor health] outcomes reflect what the system rewards. . . . The U.S. healthcare system undervalues human relationships, connections, and longitudinal primary care, unsurprisingly, it falls short. . . . Technology and human capital will need to be integrated if we are going to deliver high-quality, patient-centered care. . . . A critical challenge involves redesigning payment systems to intentionally support and provide incentives for care transformation that improves patient health and patient experience.

—Marshall H. Chin, MD[2]

These two quotes effectively summarize some of the most material problems with the U.S. health system. Why do we have these major problems? Because our approach to health reform does not focus on the root cause of our problems—the real issues driving the system. We blame administrators, unfair billing practices, or large corporations. However, these groups and systems are not at the core of the problem. My perspective is that the core problems are (1) fragmented care, which causes medical errors, destroys relationships, and is expensive; (2) a ridiculously complex billing system that creates economic incentives for fragmented care; and (3) unrealistic expectations about how long we should live, about what medicine can do for us in old age, and about how long our resources and funds for healthcare will last. These core problems are not addressed in our health reform efforts because their solutions require trade-offs.

HEALTH POLICY RECOMMENDATIONS

1. Eliminate coding and billing from PCP compensation. The use of coding and billing is inordinately time-consuming and complicated. It disincentivizes physicians from spending time talking with and listening to their patients. This payment methodology is the driving force behind fragmented healthcare. A bolder statement on this recommendation is that our nation's obsession with coding has damaged the physician–patient relationship. There is an alternative way to pay these physicians that would restore the relationship, is straightforward to administer, and supports positive incentives for physicians and patients (see chapters 12 and 13).
2. Formally designate the PCP's office as responsible for EOL care coordination and education and the completion of AHDs.
3. Modify use of the term "medical necessity" by health insurers. Specifically, all services provided by primary care offices should per se be deemed medically necessary. Similarly, all services provided by hospice and homecare entities should be deemed medically necessary. Conversely, access to a hospital ICU bed

should be deemed medically unnecessary for terminally ill patients.

4. Require Medicare recipients to complete an AHD before they can be eligible for Medicare coverage.

5. Expand and modify insurance coverage for palliative care, hospice care, and homecare with the recommendations in chapters 14 and 16. Substantial savings for supporting these expanded health benefits (although support may not be needed) will be found by taxing healthcare benefits as equivalent to wages; eliminating prescription drug advertising; and reducing excessive variation in Medicare payments according to geographic location.

6. Create national guidelines for health insurance coverage that integrate economics with clinical effectiveness. These guidelines would be developed by an independent, nonpolitical organization.

7. Offer premium discounts on Medicare Part B coverage for patients willing to complete educational videos on EOL care options. Videos have been found to be effective tools for educating and informing patients of their care options.

8. Treat ignoring a patient's AHD as a sentinel event. This would be an educational approach to heightening the importance of these documents for clinicians.

9. Reexamine the ethical standard for patient autonomy. Specifically, take into account the impact of care decisions on the patient's family, their consistency with clinical standards, and their economic sustainability.

10. Formally re-evaluate CPR and Do Not Resuscitate standards and modify the laws and practices governing their use.

11. Permanently accept telehealth as a medically necessary service and reimburse accordingly. This service has proven its value to patients and physicians.

12. Embed an AHD in every patient's electronic medical record.

13. Ensure physicians have easy access to every patient's electronic record in general, regardless of vendor. This concept is known in the health field as the interoperability of the electronic record. Knowing a patient's full history of care would be an

important step to improving the quality of patient encounters and reducing fragmented care.

14. Develop a consultation trigger for palliative care for patients over age 65 being offered services such as a transplant, a ventilator, a feeding tube, entering a clinical trial, or kidney dialysis. This consultation should include a conversation on the patient's AHD.

PERSONAL PREPARATION RECOMMENDATIONS FOR END-OF-LIFE CARE

1. Open your mind to thinking about your own death. Face your fear of death. It isn't easy. We are programmed not to think about our own death. That said, intentionally preparing for EOL care is important. Dying, like living, benefits from preparation. Assume more responsibility for determining how you wish to use healthcare in your later years. Otherwise you are implicitly accepting the death trap. Doing any task well requires effort and dying is no exception.

2. Prepare for accepting that your mental and physical capacity will decline as you age. Accepting this fundamental reality is one part of setting realistic expectations for elderhood.

3. Think about the question "Am I old enough to die?" Intentionally try to decide when you have lived a full life. Wanting more and more from life could be considered greedy. This perspective will not be a Eureka! moment but a gradual acceptance. As you begin to reach this point, consider diminishing future medical treatment and tests. Ask yourself what the costs and benefits of these care options are. The benefit of these treatments may be less than you think, and the costs may be higher than you think.

4. Complete an AHD. When doing so, seek assistance from a clinician with expertise in this area and not a lawyer. I highly recommend the compassion protocol of the Fitzpatrick sisters (see chapter 8) as a guide to help you think through the issues surrounding the completion of an AHD. Remember, the more

specific your AHD, the more helpful it will be to your family and caregivers.

5. Discuss your feelings about EOL care with the surrogate or surrogates you have named in your HCPA. Do they understand your desires? Will they be comfortable making healthcare decisions for you? Will they be available to make these decisions for you? Will they be too emotionally involved to be objective? These questions should all be part of your conversation, and it would be unfair to your surrogate or surrogates not to ask them.

6. Remember that dying is not just a clinical issue; it is a philosophy-of-life issue. Don't confuse medical advice with life advice. This is your life and you're under no obligation to keep seeking healthcare when that healthcare is no longer effective. These choices are more a question of wisdom than of medical options. Doctors are hardwired to try and keep patients alive at all costs, and patients instinctively want to live longer. The ensuing procedures lead to even more procedures, but this chain reaction of care, counterintuitively, leads to new kinds of suffering.

7. Heed this advice from Pastor Forrest Church: "Love and death are allies. When a loved one dies, the greater the pain, the greater love's proof. Such grief is a sacrament. Sacraments bring us together. The measure of our grief testifies to the power of love. . . . We cannot protect love from death. But giving away our hearts, can protect our lives from the death of love."[3]

And here's one final reflection for you and your family from Pastor Church: "The act of releasing a loved one from all further obligations as he lies dying—to tell him it's alright, that he is safe, that we love him and he can go now—is life's most perfect gift, the final expression of unconditional love."[4]

Our love for others lives forever, and this love is our life legacy.

NOTES

FOREWORD

1. Paul B. Batalden and Frank Davidoff, "What Is 'Quality Improvement' and How Can It Transform Healthcare?" *Quality & Safety in Health Care* 16, no. 1 (2007).

2. William H. Shrank, Teresa L. Rogstad, and Natasha Parekh, "Waste in the US Health Care System: Estimated Costs and Potential for Savings," *JAMA* 322, no. 15 (2019).

INTRODUCTION

1. Libby Sallnow et al., "Report of the *Lancet* Commission on the Value of Death: Bringing Death Back Into Life," *Lancet* 399, no. 10327 (February 26, 2022): 837–84.

2. Sallnow et al., "Report of the *Lancet* Commission."

CHAPTER 1

1. Uwe E. Reinhardt, *Priced Out: The Economic and Ethical Costs of American Health Care* (Princeton, NJ: Princeton University Press, 2019), 146.

2. Sohrab Ahmari, *The Unbroken Thread: Discovering the Wisdom of Tradition in an Age of Chaos* (New York: Convergent, 2021), 247.

3. Ibid., 254.

4. Ibid., 255.

5. Ibid., 257–58.

6. Ibid., 259–60.

7. The names used in the patient stories (other than those of my immediate family members) are fictitious. These stories are actual events recalled to the best of my ability.

CHAPTER 2

1. Laozi, known as "Lao Tzu," was an ancient Chinese philosopher and writer from the sixth century BCE. He is considered the founder of philosophical Taoism and was a contemporary of Confucius.

2. Ann Neumann, *The Good Death: An Exploration of Dying in America* (Boston: Beacon Press, 2016), 8.

3. Leslie J. Blackhall, "Must We Always Use CPR?" *New England Journal of Medicine* 317, no. 20 (1987).

4. Ibid.

5. Ibid.

6. Ibid.

7. Ibid.

8. Kenneth A. Fisher, Lindsay E. Rockwell, and Missy Scott, *In Defiance of Death: Exposing the Real Costs of End-of-Life Care* (Westport, CT: Praeger, 2008), 18.

9. Jeanne Fitzpatrick and Eileen Fitzpatrick, *A Better Way of Dying: How to Make the Best Choices at the End of Life* (New York: Penguin Books, 2010), 97.

10. Ibid.

11. L. S. Dugdale, *The Lost Art of Dying: Reviving Forgotten Wisdom* (New York: HarperCollins, 2020), 97–99.

12. "Death Panels" is a political term that originated in the 2009 debate over federal healthcare legislation (Obama Care) to cover the uninsured in the United States. Sarah Palin, governor of Alaska and vice presidential candidate in 2008, coined the term when she charged that the proposed legislation would create death panels of bureaucrats who would carry out triage.

13. CMS Medicare Learning Network, "MLN Fact Sheet: Advance Care Center for Medicare & Medicaid Services Planning," 2020. "Voluntary ACP" is a face-to-face service between a Medicare physician (or other qualified healthcare professional) and a patient to discuss the patient's wishes if they become unable to make decisions about their care. This is a Medicare Part B service billed under CPT codes 99497 and 99498.

14. American Medical Association, "Code of Medical Ethics Overview," www.ama-assn.org/delivering-care/ethics/code-medical-ethics-overview. The 2001 revision of "Principles of Medical Ethics" added two new prin-

ciples. One emphasizes that a physician, while caring for a patient, should regard responsibility to the patient as paramount.

15. Jessica Nutik Zitter, *Extreme Measures: Finding a Better Path to the End of Life* (New York: Avery, 2017), 69.

CHAPTER 3

1. Yair Dor-Ziderman, Antoine Lutz, and Abraham Goldstein, "Prediction-Based Neural Mechanisms for Shielding the Self from Existential Threat," *NeuroImage* 202 (2019).

2. Ibid.

3. Neumann, *The Good Death*, 12.

4. Lynda Gratton and Andrew Scott, *The 100-Year Life: Living and Working in an Age of Longevity* (London: Bloomsbury Publishing, 2016), 79.

5. Sallnow et al., "Report of the Lancet Commission."

6. Barbara Ehrenreich, *Natural Causes: An Epidemic of Wellness, the Certainty of Dying and Killing Ourselves to Live Longer* (New York: Twelve, 2018), xv.

7. Ibid., 3.

8. Ibid.

9. Ibid.

10. Ibid.

11. Kuldeep N. Yadav et al., "Approximately One in Three US Adults Completes Any Type of Advance Directive for End-of-Life Care," *Health Aff (Millwood)* 36, no. 7 (2017).

12. Paula Span, "For Older Patients, an 'Afterworld' of Hospital Care," *New York Times* 2019.

13. Ibid.

14. Ibid.

15. Ibid.

16. Ibid.

17. Ibid.

CHAPTER 4

1. Peter Manseau, *The Jefferson Bible: A Biography* (Princeton, NJ: Princeton University Press, 2020), 19.

2. Jason M. Baxter, *The Medieval Mind of C. S. Lewis: How Great Books Shaped a Great Mind* (Downers Grove, IL: IVP Academic, 2022), 62.

3. Ibid., 66–67.

4. Thomas Krystofiak, *Tempted to Believe: The Seduction of the Promise of Certainty* (Self-published, 2020), 50.

5. Ibid., 59.

6. Abraham Flexner, "Medical Education in the United States and Canada: A Report to the Carnegie Foundation for the Advancement of Teaching," Carnegie Foundation, 1910.

7. Dr. David Leach, email message to author, January 21, 2021.

8. Charles C. Camosy, *Losing Our Dignity: How Secularized Medicine Is Undermining Fundamental Human Equity* (Hyde Park, NY: New City Press, 2021).

9. Ibid.

10. Ludwig Edelstein, *The Hippocratic Oath, Text, Translation and Interpretation* (Baltimore, MD: Johns Hopkins University Press, 1943).

11. Jonatan Pallesen, June 9, 2019.

12. Louise Aronson, *Elderhood: Redefining Aging, Transforming Medicine, Reimagining Life* (New York: Bloomsbury Publishing, 2019), 136.

13. Ibid.

14. Ibid.

15. Ibid.

16. Henry D. Thoreau, *The Writings of Henry Thoreau, Vol. 1* (New York: Houghton and Mifflin, 1893), 125.

CHAPTER 5

1. Kimberly Amadeo, "US Budget Deficit by Year Compared to GDP, the National Debt, and Events," The Balance, www.thebalance.com/us-deficit-by-year-3306306.

2. Louise Sheiner, "The Long-Term Impact of Aging on the Federal Budget" (Washington, DC: Brookings Institution, 2018).

3. Ibid.

4. Harry Robertson, "Almost a Fifth of All US Dollars Were Created This Year," City A.M., www.cityam.com/almost-a-fifth-of-all-us-dollars-were-created-this-year/.

5. Rebecca L. Clark et al., "Federal Expenditures on Children: 1960–1997" (Washington, DC: Urban Institute, 2001).

6. Peter G. Peterson Foundation, "How Much Government Spending Goes to Children?" www.pgpf.org/blog/2022/01/how-much-government-spending-goes-to-children.

7. Ibid.; Sheiner, "The Long-Term Impact."

8. Anne B. Martin et al., "National Health Care Spending in 2019: Steady Growth for the Fourth Consecutive Year," *Health Affairs* 40, no. 1 (2020).

9. Ian Duncan et al., "Medicare Cost at End of Life," *American Journal of Hospice and Palliative Medicine* 36, no. 8 (2019).

10. Ibid.

11. Ibid.

12. Ibid.

13. Gerald F. Riley and James D. Lubitz, "Long-Term Trends in Medicare Payments in the Last Year of Life," *Health Services Research* 45, no. 2 (2010).

14. Ibid.

15. Ibid.

16. Ibid.

17. Liran Einav et al., "Predictive Modeling of U.S. Health Care Spending in Late Life," *Science* 360, no. 6396 (2018).

18. Angelo E. Volandes, *The Conversation: A Revolutionary Plan for End-of-Life Care* (New York: Bloomsbury Publishing, 2015).

19. Ibid.

20. Issues Committee on Approaching Death, "Dying in America: Improving Quality and Honoring Individual Preferences near the End of Life" (Washington, DC: National Academies Press, 2015), 8–9.

21. Medicare Payment Advisory Committee, "Report to the Congress: Medicare and the Health Care Delivery Sysyem," 2015.

22. Centers for Medicare & Medicaid Services, "National Health Expenditure Projections 2021–30: Moderate as COVID-19 Impacts Wane," 2022.

23. CBS News, Los Angeles, "Medicare to Become Insolvent in 2026, Three Years Earlier Than Forecast," June 5, 2018.

24. Joanne Lynn, *Medicaring Communities: Getting What We Want and Need in Frail Old Age at an Affordable Price* (Ann Arbor, MI: Altarum Institute, 2016), 8.

25. Ibid., 15.

26. Stephen J. Dubner, "Are You Ready for a Glorius Sunset?" Freakonomics Radio 40:55, 2015.

27. Ibid.

28. Ibid.

29. Ibid.

30. Ibid.

31. Ibid.

32. Ezekial Emanuel, "My 92-Year-Old Father Didn't Need More Medical Care," *Alantic Monthly*, January 2, 2020.

33. Ibid.

34. Ibid.

35. Ibid.

CHAPTER 6

1. Daniela J. Lamas, "Who Are We Caring for in the I.C.U.?" *New York Times*, 2022.

2. David Weissman, "Policy Proposal: Do Not Resuscitate Orders: A Call for Reform," *Virtual Mentor* 5, no. 1 (2003).

3. Ibid.

4. Ibid.

5. Ibid.

6. Leeat Granek, "When Doctors Grieve," *New York Times*, May 25, 2012.

7. Ibid.

8. Ibid.

9. Ibid.

10. Ibid.

11. Katy Butler, "Preparing for a Good End of Life," *Wall Street Journal*, February 8, 2019.

12. Atul Gawande, *Being Mortal: Medicine and What Matters in the End* (New York: Metropolitan Books, 2014), 1.

13. Atul Gawande, "Letting Go," *New Yorker*, August 2, 2010.

14. Ibid.

15. Ibid.

16. Ibid.

17. Ibid.

18. Ibid.

19. Neumann, *The Good Death*.

20. Stephen J. Dubner, "Are You Ready for a Glorious Sunset?," Freakonomics Radio 40:55, 2015.

21. Daniel P. Sulmasy, "Holding Life and Death in Dynamic Tension," *Health Progress* (2017): 32.

22. Ibid.

23. Ibid.

24. Sallie Tisdale, *Advice for Future Corpses (and Those Who Love Them): A Practical Perspective on Death and Dying* (New York: Touchstone, 2018), 120–21.

CHAPTER 7

1. Marcella Alsan, Marianne Wanamaker, and Rachel R. Hardeman, "The Tuskegee Study of Untreated Syphilis: A Case Study in Peripheral Trauma with Implications for Health Professionals," *Journal of General Internal Medicine* 35, no. 1 (2020).

2. Dale Hardy et al., "Racial Disparities in the Use of Hospice Services According to Geographic Residence and Socioeconomic Status in an Elderly Cohort with Nonsmall Cell Lung Cancer," *Cancer* 117, no. 7 (2011); Lilian Liou Cohen, "Racial/Ethnic Disparities in Hospice Care: A Systematic Review," *Journal of Palliative Medicine* 11, no. 5 (2008).

3. Centers for Disease Control and Prevention, "Health Equity Considerations and Racial and Ethnic Minority Groups," https://www.cdc.gov /coronavirus/2019-ncov/community/health-equity/race-ethnicity.html.

4. Danielle M. Ely and Anne K. Driscoll, "Infant Mortality in the United States, 2018: Data from the Period Linked Birth/Infant Death File," in *National Vital Statistics Reports* (Center for Disease Control and Prevention, 2020).

5. John J. Paris, "Catholic Approaches to End-of-Life Care," *America*, September 22, 2015.

6. Ibid.

7. Ibid.

8. Ibid.

9. Sophie Evans, "Alfie Evans' Condition: Brain Disease Which Was So Tricky to Diagnose and Has No Name," *Mirror*, April 28, 2018.

10. Betsy McCaughey, "Pulling the Plug against Parents' Wishes," *New York Post*, April 25, 2018.

11. Ibid.

12. *Nancy Beth Cruzan, by Her Parents and Co-Guardians, Cruzan et Ux. V. Director, Missouri Department of Health, et al.*, (1990).

13. M. K. Robinson, M. J. DeHaven, and K. A. Koch, "Effects of the Patient Self-Determination Act on Patient Knowledge and Behavior," *Journal of Family Practice* 37, no. 4 (1993).

14. Jake Zuckerman and Terry DeMio, "Judge Rules Hospital Must Use Ivermectin: COVID–19 Patient Sought Drug CDC Warns Against," *Cincinnati Enquirer*, August 31, 2021; Cameron Knight, "Judge Rules Hospital Cannot Be Forced to Give Ivermectin," *Cincinnati Enquirer*, September 8, 2021.

CHAPTER 8

1. Elisabeth Kübler-Ross, *On Death and Dying* (New York: Macmillan, 1969).

2. Ibid., 262.

3. Ernest Becker, *The Denial of Death* (New York: Free Press, 1973), xvii.

4. Ibid.

5. Ibid.

6. Ibid., xiii.

7. Sheldon Solomon, Jeff Greenberg, and Tom Pyszczynski, *The Worm at the Core: On the Role of Death in Life* (New York: Random House, 2015), xi.

8. Ibid., 87–88.

9. Ibid., 81.

10. Jeanne Fitzpatrick and Eileen Fitzpatrick, *A Better Way of Dying: How to Make the Best Choices at the End of Life* (New York: Penguin Books, 2010), 16.

11. Ibid., 5.

12. Ibid.

13. Ibid., 209–14.

14. Dr. David Leach, email message to author, August 19, 2021.

CHAPTER 9

1. Solveig Hauge and Heggen Kristin, "The Nursing Home as a Home: A Field Study of Residents' Daily Life in the Common Living Rooms," *Journal of Clinical Nursing* 17, no. 4 (2008).

2. Joseph E. Davis, "No Country for Old Age," *Hedgehog Review* (2018).

3. Thomas R. Cole and Mary G. Winkler, eds., *The Oxford Book of Aging* (Oxford: Oxford University Press, 1994), 4.

4. Ecclesiastes 3:1 (KJV).

5. Marcus Tullius Cicero, *How to Grow Old: Ancient Wisdom for the Second Half of Life*, trans. Philip Freeman (Princeton, NJ: Princeton University Press, 2016), xiii.

6. Ibid.

7. Ibid., xiv–xv.

8. Walter Nicgorski, "Cicero and the Natural Law" (2011).

9. Arthur C. Brooks, "Your Professional Decline Is Coming (Much) Sooner Than You Think," *Atlantic*, July 2019.

10. Ibid.

11. Ibid.

12. Ibid.

CHAPTER 10

1. Joanne Lynn, *Medicaring Communities: Getting What We Want and Need in Frail Old Age at an Affordable Price* (Altarum Institute, 2016), 77.

2. Ibid., 118.

3. Ibid., 108–9.

4. National Institute of Aging, "What Are Palliative Care and Hospice Care?" www.nia.nih.gov/health/what-are-palliative-care-and-hospice-care.

5. Ibid.

6. Ibid.

7. Caroline Richmond, "Dame Cicely Saunders," *British Medical Journal* 331, no. 7510 (2005).

8. John Hughes, "UK: The Best Place in the World to Die," *British Medical Journal* 351 (2015).

9. Katy Butler, *The Art of Dying Well: A Practical Guide to a Good End of Life* (New York: Scribner, 2019), 9.

10. Ezekiel J. Emanuel et al., "Attitudes and Practices of Euthanasia and Physician-Assisted Suicide in the United States, Canada, and Europe," *JAMA* 316, no. 1 (2016).

11. Pope Francis, *The Name of God Is Mercy*, trans. Oonagh Stransky (New York: Random House, 2016).

12. G. K. Chesterton, *Illustrated London News*, May 5, 1928.

CHAPTER 11

1. Amanda Singleton, "What to Know at the Beginning of Your Care Giving Journey," AARP.

2. Ibid.

3. Anne Wilkinson, Neil S. Wenger, and Lisa R. Shugarman, "Advance Directives and Advance Care Planning: Report to Congress" (U.S. Department of Health and Human Services, 2008).

4. *Nancy Beth Cruzan, by Her Parents and Co-Guardians, Cruzan et ux. v. Director, Missouri Department of Health, et al.* (1990).

5. Ibid.

6. Susan Stefan, *Rational Suicide, Irrational Laws: Examining Current Approaches to Suicide in Policy and Law* (New York: Oxford University Press, 2016), 29.

7. Tamar Lewin, "Nancy Cruzan Dies, Outlived by a Debate Over the Right to Die," *New York Times*, December 27, 1990.

8. Ibid.

9. Ibid.

10. Thomas D. Harter, "What Kind of Advance Care Planning Should CMS Pay For?" Health Affairs. https://www.healthaffairs.org/do/10.1377/forefront.20150319.045549.

11. Ibid.

12. David Watkins, "Advance Care Planning and Its Impact on Surviving Family Members (and Hospitals)," Mather Institute.

13. Ibid.

14. Bernard J. Hammes and Brenda L. Rooney, "Death and End-of-Life Planning in One Midwestern Community," *Archives of Internal Medicine* 158, no. 4 (1998).

15. Ibid.

16. "Wisconsin State Profile" (State Health Access Data Assistance Center, 2015).

CHAPTER 12

1. Sarah Kliff, "COVID Killed His Father: Then Came $1 Million in Medical Bills," *New York Times*, May 21, 2021.

2. Ibid.

3. Ibid.

4. Ibid.

5. Danielle Ofri, "The Patients vs. Paperwork Problem for Doctors," *New York Times*, November 14, 2017.

6. Ibid.

7. J. Bensing, "Doctor-Patient Communication and the Quality of Care," *Social Science Medicine* 32, no. 11 (1991).

8. David Belk, HuffPost, March 13, 2014.

9. Donald E. Casey Jr et al., "Controlling High Blood Pressure: An Evidence-Based Blueprint for Change," *American Journal of Medical Quality* 37, no. 1 (2022).

10. Ibid.

11. Shannon Brownlee, *Overtreated: Why Too Much Medicine Is Making Us Sicker and Poorer* (New York: Bloomsbury Publishing, 2008), 5.

12. Ibid., 154.

13. Sarah L. Taubman et al., "Medicaid Increases Emergency-Department Use: Evidence from Oregon's Health Insurance Experiment," *Science* 343, no. 6168 (2014).

14. Kenneth Frumkin, "How to Be Safe During (and After) Emergency Room Visits," *AARP Bulletin*, May 19, 2021.

15. Ibid.

16. Ibid.

17. Meghan O'Rourke, *The Invisible Kingdom: Reimagining Chronic Illness* (New York: Riverhead Books, 2022), 73–80.

18. Kyna Fong, "The U.S. Health Care System Isn't Built for Primary Care," *Harvard Business Review*, September 28, 2021.

CHAPTER 13

1. J. Altschuler et al., "Estimating a Reasonable Patient Panel Size for Primary Care Physicians with Team-Based Task Delegation," *Annuals of Family Medicine* 10, no. 5 (2012).

2. Louise Norris, "What Is Direct Primary Care?" Dotdash Media, www .verywellhealth.com/what-is-direct-primary-care-4777328.

3. Jennifer Thompson, email to author, March 11, 2019.

4. Doctor-Salaries.com, "Primary Care Physician Salary," www.doctor-salaries.com/physician-salary/primary-care-physician-salary.

5. Christine M. Everett et al., "Physician Assistants and Nurse Practitioners as a Usual Source of Care," *Journal of Rural Health* 25, no. 4 (2009).

CHAPTER 14

1. Jessica Nutik Zitter, *Extreme Measures: Finding a Better Path to the End of Life* (New York: Avery, 2017), 54.

2. Ibid.

3. Ibid.

4. Keith Kranker et al., "Evaluation of the Medicare Care Choices Model: Annual Report 4" (Mathematica, 2022).

5. Ibid.

6. David Maichese, "Covid Has Traumatized America—a Doctor Explains What We Need to Heal," *New York Times*, March 24, 2022.

7. Ibid.

8. Sallie Tisdale, *Advice for Future Corpses (and Those Who Love Them): A Practical Perspective on Death and Dying* (New York: Touchstone, 2018), 98.

9. Ibid.

CHAPTER 15

1. Jonathan Gruber, "The Tax Exclusion for Employer-Sponsored Health Insurance," *National Tax Journal* 64, no. 2.2 (2011).
2. Uwe E. Reinhardt, *Priced Out: The Economic and Ethical Costs of American Health Care* (Princeton, NJ: Princeton University Press, 2019).
3. C. Lee Ventola, "Direct-to-Consumer Pharmaceutical Advertising: Therapeutic or Toxic?" *P&T* 36, no. 10 (2011): 671.
4. G. A. Abel et al., "Direct-to-Consumer Advertising in Oncology," *Oncologist* 11, no. 2 (2006).
5. United States Government Accountability Office, "Prescription Drugs: Medicare Spending on Drugs with Direct-to-Consumer Advertising" (2021).
6. Knowledge at Wharton, "Cause and Effect: Do Prescription Drug Ads Really Work?" https://knowledge.wharton.upenn.edu/article/prescription-drug-ads.
7. Abby E. Alpert, Neeraj Sood, and Darius N. Lakdawalla, "Prescription Drug Advertising and Drug Utilization: The Role of Medicare Part D" (2015).
8. Patrick Radden Keefe, *Empire of Pain: The Secret History of the Sackler Dynasty* (New York: Doubleday, 2021). Beth Macy, *Dopesick: Dealers, Doctors, and the Drug Company That Addicted America* (Boston: Little and Brown, 2018).
9. D. Lassman et al., "Health Spending by State 1991–2014: Measuring Per Capita Spending by Payers and Programs," *Health Affairs* 36, no. 7 (2017).
10. Lassman et al., "Health Spending by State 1991–2014."

CHAPTER 16

1. Matthew J. Press, "Instant Replay: A Quarterback's View of Care Coordination," *New England Journal of Medicine* 371, no. 6 (2014): 489.
2. Ibid.
3. Vipul Bhatia et al., "Systemwide Advance Care Planning During the Covid-19 Pandemic: The Impact on Patient Outcomes and Cost," *NEJM Catalyst* 2, no. 9 (2021): 9.
4. Joan M. Teno, "Promoting Multifaceted Interventions for Care of the Seriously Ill and Dying," *JAMA Health Forum* 3, no. 4 (2022): 1.
5. Ibid., 3.
6. Atul Gawande, "Letting Go," *New Yorker*, August 2, 2010.
7. Angelo E. Volandes, *The Conversation: A Revolutionary Plan for End-of-Life Care* (New York: Bloomsbury, 2015).

CHAPTER 17

1. Freakonomics Radio, "Is Dialysis a Test Case of Medicare for All?" 57:18, 2021.

2. Madalina Garbi, "National Institute for Health and Care Excellence Clinical Guidelines Development Principles and Processes," *Heart* 107, no. 12 (2021): 951.

3. Michael D. Connelly and Lawrence D. Prybil, "Charting a Course to Community Health: A Governance Priority," *Health Progress* 98, no. 5 (2017).

CHAPTER 18

1. Richard Rohr, "Coming to Terms with Life and Love," Center for Action and Contemplation.

2. Tiffany Green and Atheendar S. Venkataramani, "Trade-Offs and Policy Options—Using Insights from Economics to Inform Public Health Policy," *New England Journal of Medicine* 386, no. 5 (2022): 405.

3. Thomas Sowell, *Dismantling America: And Other Controversial Essays* (New York: Basic Books, 2010), 340.

4. Uwe E. Reinhardt, *Priced Out: The Economic and Ethical Costs of American Health Care* (Princeton, NJ: Princeton University Press, 2019), 147.

5. Eric Weiner, *The Socrates Express: In Search of Life Lessons from Dead Philosophers* (New York: Avid Reader Press, 2020), 281–82.

6. Sohrab Ahmari, *The Unbroken Thread: Discovering the Wisdom of Tradition in an Age of Chaos* (New York: Convergent, 2021).

7. Alexander Solzhenitsyn, "Harvard Address," 1978.

8. Ibid.

CHAPTER 19

1. Sallnow et al., "Report of the *Lancet* Commission on the Value of Death: Bringing Death Back Into Life," *Lancet* 399, no. 10327 (February 26, 2022): 30.

2. Meghan O'Rourke, *The Invisible Kingdom: Reimagining Chronic Illness* (New York: Riverhead Books, 2022).

3. Ross Douthat, *The Deep Places: A Memoir of Illness and Discovery* (New York: Convergent Books, 2021).

4. Paul W. Gleason, "The Lesson of a Long Illness: On Ross Douthat's *The Deep Places*," *Los Angeles Review of Books*, October 17, 2021.

5. Sinclair Lewis, *Arrowsmith* (New York: Harcourt Brace & Co., 1925).

6. Douthat, *The Deep Places*, 40.

7. O'Rourke, *The Invisible Kingdom*, 44.

8. Ibid., 130.

9. Anthony T. Kronman, *After Disbelief: On Disenchantment, Disappointment, Eternity, and Joy* (New Haven, CT: Yale University Press, 2022), 23.

APPENDIX

1. Quoted in Alana Newhouse, "Everything Is Broken," Tablet Magazine, January 14, 2021.

2. "Uncomfortable Truths—What COVID–19 Has Revealed About Chronic Disease in America," *New England Journal of Medicine* (October 28, 2021).

3. Forrest Church, *Love & Death: My Journey Through the Valley of the Shadow* (Boston: Beacon Press, 2008), 10–11.

4. Ibid.

BIBLIOGRAPHY

Abel, G. A., R. T. Penson, S. Joffe, L. Schapira, B. A. Chabner, and T. J. Lynch Jr. "Direct-to-Consumer Advertising in Oncology." *Oncologist* 11, no. 2 (February 2006): 217–26.

Ahmari, Sohrab. *The Unbroken Thread: Discovering the Wisdom of Tradition in an Age of Chaos.* New York: Convergent, 2021.

Alpert, Abby E., Neeraj Sood, and Darius N. Lakdawalla. "Prescription Drug Advertising and Drug Utilization: The Role of Medicare Part D." (2015).

Alsan, Marcella, Marianne Wanamaker, and Rachel R. Hardeman. "The Tuskegee Study of Untreated Syphilis: A Case Study in Peripheral Trauma with Implications for Health Professionals." *Journal of General Internal Medicine* 35, no. 1 (2020): 322–25.

Altschuler, J., D. Margolius, T. Bodenheimer, and K. Grumbach. "Estimating a Reasonable Patient Panel Size for Primary Care Physicians with Team-Based Task Delegation." *Annuals of Family Medicine* 10, no. 5 (September–October 2012): 396–400.

Amadeo, Kimberly. "US Budget Deficit by Year Compared to GDP, the National Debt, and Events." The Balance, www.thebalance.com/us-deficit-by -year-3306306.

Aronson, Louise. *Elderhood: Redefining Aging, Transforming Medicine, Reimagining Life.* New York: Bloomsbury Publishing, 2019.

Batalden, Paul B., and Frank Davidoff. "What Is "Quality Improvement" and How Can It Transform Healthcare?" *Quality & Safety in Health Care* 16, no. 1 (2007): 2–3.

Baxter, Jason M. *The Medieval Mind of C. S. Lewis: How Great Books Shaped a Great Mind.* Downers Grove, IL: IVP Academic, 2022.

Becker, Ernest. *The Denial of Death.* New York: Free Press, 1973.

Belk, David. "Dependence Through Denial and Deception: How Health Insurance Companies Keep Your Premiums High." HuffPost, 2014.

Bensing, J. "Doctor-Patient Communication and the Quality of Care." *Social Science Medicine* 32, no. 11 (1991): 1301–10.

Bhatia, Vipul, Roberta Geidner, Kamna Mirchandani, Yue Huang, and Haider J. Warraich. "Systemwide Advance Care Planning During the COVID-19 Pandemic: The Impact on Patient Outcomes and Cost." *NEJM Catalyst* 2, no. 9 (2021).

Blackhall, Leslie J. "Must We Always Use CPR?" *New England Journal of Medicine* 317, no. 20 (1987): 1281–85.

Brooks, Arthur C. "Your Professional Decline Is Coming (Much) Sooner Than You Think." *Atlantic*, July 2019.

Brownlee, Shannon. *Overtreated: Why Too Much Medicine Is Making Us Sicker and Poorer.* New York: Bloomsbury Publishing, 2008.

Butler, Katy. *The Art of Dying Well: A Practical Guide to a Good End of Life.* New York: Scribner, 2019.

———. "Preparing for a Good End of Life." *Wall Street Journal*, February 8, 2019.

Camosy, Charles C. *Losing Our Dignity: How Secularized Medicine Is Undermining Fundamental Human Equity.* Hyde Park, NY: New City Press, 2021.

Casey, Donald E. Jr, Donna M. Daniel, Jay Bhatt, Robert M. Carey, Yvonne Commodore-Mensah, Aline Holmes, Alison P. Smith, Gregory Wozniak, and Jackson T. Wright Jr. "Controlling High Blood Pressure: An Evidence-Based Blueprint for Change." *American Journal of Medical Quality* 37, no. 1 (2022): 22–31.

CBS. "Medicare to Become Insolvent in 2026, Three Years Earlier Than Forecast." June 5, 2018.

Centers for Disease Control and Prevention. "Health Equity Considerations and Racial and Ethnic Minority Groups." www.cdc.gov/coronavirus/2019 -ncov/community/health-equity/race-ethnicity.html.

Centers for Medicare & Medicaid Services. "National Health Expenditure Projections 2021–30: Moderate as COVID–19 Impacts Wane," 2022.

———. "MLN Fact Sheet: Advance Care Planning," 2020.

Chesterton, G. K. *Illustrated London News*, May 5, 1928.

Church, Forrest. *Love & Death: My Journey Through the Valley of the Shadow.* Boston: Beacon Press, 2008.

Cicero, Marcus Tullius. *How to Grow Old: Ancient Wisdom for the Second Half of Life.* Translated by Philip Freeman. Princeton, NJ: Princeton University Press, 2016.

Clark, Rebecca L., Rosalind Berkowitz King, Christopher Spiro, and C. Eugene Steuerle. "Federal Expenditures on Children: 1960–1997." Washington, DC: Urban Institute, 2001.

Cohen, Lilian Liou. "Racial/Ethnic Disparities in Hospice Care: A Systematic Review." *Journal of Palliative Medicine* 11, no. 5 (2008): 763–68.

Cole, Thomas R., and Mary G. Winkler, eds. *The Oxford Book of Aging*. Oxford: Oxford University Press, 1994.

Committee on Approaching Death: Addressing Key End of Life, Issues, and Institute of Medicine. "Dying in America: Improving Quality and Honoring Individual Preferences Near the End of Life." Washington, DC: National Academies Press, 2015.

Connelly, Michael D., and D. Prybil Lawrence. "Charting a Course to Community Health: A Governance Priority." *Health Progress* 98, no. 5 (2017): 71.

Davis, Joseph E. "No Country for Old Age." *Hedgehog Review* (2018).

Doctor Salaries, "Primary Care Physician Salary." www.doctor-salaries.com /physician-salary/primary-care-physician-salary.

Dor-Ziderman, Yair, Antoine Lutz, and Abraham Goldstein. "Prediction-Based Neural Mechanisms for Shielding the Self from Existential Threat." *NeuroImage* 202 (November 15, 2019): 116080.

Douthat, Ross. *The Deep Places: A Memoir of Illness and Discovery*. New York: Convergent Books, 2021.

Dubner, Stephen J. *Are You Ready for a Glorious Sunset?* Freakonomics Radio 40:55, 2015.

Dugdale, L. S. *The Lost Art of Dying: Reviving Forgotten Wisdom*. New York: HarperCollins, 2020.

Duncan, Ian, Tamim Ahmed, Henry Dove, and Terri L. Maxwell. "Medicare Cost at End of Life." *American Journal of Hospice and Palliative Medicine* 36, no. 8 (2019): 705–10.

Edelstein, Ludwig. *The Hippocratic Oath, Text, Translation and Interpretation*. Baltimore, MD: Johns Hopkins University Press, 1943.

Ehrenreich, Barbara. *Natural Causes: An Epidemic of Wellness, the Certainty of Dying and Killing Ourselves to Live Longer*. New York: Twelve, 2018.

Einav, Liran, Amy Finkelstein, Sendhil Mullainathan, and Ziad Obermeyer. "Predictive Modeling of U.S. Health Care Spending in Late Life." *Science* 360, no. 6396 (2018): 1462–65.

Ely, Danielle M., and Anne K. Driscoll. "Infant Mortality in the United States, 2018: Data from the Period Linked Birth/Infant Death File." In *National Vital Statistics Reports*: Center for Disease Control and Prevention, 2020.

Emanuel, Ezekial. "My 92-Year-Old Father Didn't Need More Medical Care." *Atlantic*, January 2, 2020.

Emanuel, Ezekiel J., Bregje D. Onwuteaka-Philipsen, John W. Urwin, and Joachim Cohen. "Attitudes and Practices of Euthanasia and Physician-

Assisted Suicide in the United States, Canada, and Europe." *JAMA* 316, no. 1 (2016): 79–90.

Evans, Sophie. "Alfie Evans' Condition: Brain Disease Which Was So Tricky to Diagnose and Has No Name." *Mirror*, April 28, 2018.

Everett, Christine M., Jessica R. Schumacher, Alexandra Wright, and Maureen A. Smith. "Physician Assistants and Nurse Practitioners as a Usual Source of Care." *Journal of Rural Health* 25, no. 4 (2009): 407–14.

Fisher, Kenneth A., Lindsay E. Rockwell, and Missy Scott. *In Defiance of Death: Exposing the Real Costs of End-of-Life Care*. Westport, CT: Praeger, 2008.

Fitzpatrick, Jeanne, and Eileen Fitzpatrick. *A Better Way of Dying: How to Make the Best Choices at the End of Life*. New York: Penguin Books, 2010.

Flexner, Abraham. "Medical Education in the United States and Canada: A Report to the Carnegie Foundation for the Advancement of Teaching." New York: Carnegie Foundation, 1910.

Fong, Kyna. "The U.S. Health Care System Isn't Built for Primary Care." *Harvard Business Review*, September 28, 2021.

Francis, Pope. *The Name of God Is Mercy*. Translated by Oonagh Stransky. New York: Random House, 2016.

Freakonomics Radio. "Is Dialysis a Test Case of Medicare for All?" 57:18, 2021.

Frumkin, Kenneth. "How to Be Safe During (and After) Emergency Room Visits." *AARP Bulletin*, May 19, 2021.

Garbi, Madalina. "National Institute for Health and Care Excellence Clinical Guidelines Development Principles and Processes." *Heart* 107, no. 12 (2021): 949–53.

Gawande, Atul. *Being Mortal: Medicine and What Matters in the End*. New York: Metropolitan Books, 2014.

———. "Letting Go." *New Yorker*, August 2, 2010.

Gleason, Paul W. "The Lesson of a Long Illness: On Ross Douthat's 'The Deep Places.'" *Los Angeles Review of Books*, October 17, 2021.

Granek, Leeat. "When Doctors Grieve." *New York Times*, May 25, 2012.

Gratton, Lynda, and Andrew Scott. *The 100-Year Life: Living and Working in an Age of Longevity*. London: Bloomsbury Publishing, 2016.

Green, Tiffany, and Atheendar S. Venkataramani. "Trade-Offs and Policy Options—Using Insights from Economics to Inform Public Health Policy." *New England Journal of Medicine* 386, no. 5 (2022): 405–8.

Gruber, Jonathan. "The Tax Exclusion for Employer-Sponsored Health Insurance." *National Tax Journal* 64, no. 2.2 (2011): 511–30.

Hammes, Bernard J., and Brenda L. Rooney. "Death and End-of-Life Planning in One Midwestern Community." *Archives of Internal Medicine* 158, no. 4 (1998): 383–90.

Hardy, Dale, Wenyaw Chan, Chih-Chin Liu, Janice N. Cormier, Rui Xia, Eduardo Bruera, and Xianglin L. Du. "Racial Disparities in the Use of Hospice Services According to Geographic Residence and Socioeconomic Status in an Elderly Cohort with Nonsmall Cell Lung Cancer." *Cancer* 117, no. 7 (2011): 1506–15.

Harter, Thomas D. "What Kind of Advance Care Planning Should CMS Pay For?" Health Affairs. www.healthaffairs.org/do/10.1377/forefront.20150319.045549.

Hauge, Solveig, and Heggen Kristin. "The Nursing Home as a Home: A Field Study of Residents' Daily Life in the Common Living Rooms." *Journal of Clinical Nursing* 17, no. 4 (2008): 460–67.

Hughes, John. "UK: The Best Place in the World to Die." *British Medical Journal* 351 (2015): h5440.

Keefe, Patrick Radden. *Empire of Pain: The Secret History of the Sackler Dynasty.* New York: Doubleday, 2021.

Kliff, Sarah. "COVID Killed His Father. Then Came $1 Million in Medical Bills." *New York Times*, May 21, 2021.

Knight, Cameron. "Judge Rules Hospital Cannot Be Forced to Give Ivermectin." *Cincinnati Enquirer*, September 8, 2021.

Kranker, Keith, Matthew Niedzwiecki, R. Vincent Pohl, Arnold Chen, Marlena Luhr, Lauren Vollmer Forrow, and Valerie Cheh. "Evaluation of the Medicare Care Choices Model: Annual Report 4." *Mathematica*, 2022.

Kronman, Anthony T. *After Disbelief: On Disenchantment, Disappointment, Eternity, and Joy.* New Haven, CT: Yale University Press, 2022.

Krystofiak, Thomas. "Tempted to Believe: The Seduction of the Promise of Certainty." Self-published, 2020.

Kübler-Ross, Elisabeth. *On Death and Dying.* New York: Macmillan, 1969.

Lamas, Daniela J. "Who Are We Caring for in the I.C.U.?" *New York Times*, 2022.

Lassman, D., A. M. Sisko, A. Catlin, M. C. Barron, J. Benson, G. A. Cuckler, M. Hartman, A. B. Martin, and L. Whittle. "Health Spending by State 1991–2014: Measuring Per Capita Spending by Payers and Programs." *Health Affairs* 36, no. 7 (July 1, 2017): 1318–27.

Lewin, Tamar. "Nancy Cruzan Dies, Outlived by a Debate Over the Right to Die." *New York Times*, December 27, 1990.

Lewis, Sinclair. *Arrowsmith.* New York: Harcourt Brace & Co., 1925.

Lynn, Joanne. *Medicaring Communities: Getting What We Want and Need in Frail Old Age at an Affordable Price.* Altarum Institute, 2016.

Macy, Beth. *Dopesick: Dealers, Doctors, and the Drug Company That Addicted America.* Boston: Little and Brown, 2018.

Maichese, David. "COVID Has Traumatized America—A Doctor Explains What We Need to Heal." *New York Times*, March 24, 2022.

Manseau, Peter. *The Jefferson Bible: A Biography*. Princeton, NJ: Princeton University Press, 2020.

Martin, Anne B., Micah Hartman, David Lassman, and Aaron Catlin. "National Health Care Spending in 2019: Steady Growth for the Fourth Consecutive Year." *Health Affairs* 40, no. 1 (December 16, 2020): 14–24.

McCaughey, Betsy. "Pulling the Plug Against Parents' Wishes." *New York Post*, April 25, 2018.

MedPAC. "Report to Congress: Medicare and the Health Care Delivery System," 2015.

Nancy Beth Cruzan, by Her Parents and Co-Guardians, Cruzan Et Ux. V. Director, Missouri Department of Health, Et Al. (1990).

National Institute of Aging, "What Are Palliative Care and Hospice Care?" www.nia.nih.gov/health/what-are-palliative-care-and-hospice-care.

Neumann, Ann. *The Good Death: An Exploration of Dying in America*. Boston: Beacon Press, 2016.

Nicgorski, Walter. "Cicero and the Natural Law." 2011.

Norris, Louise. "What Is Direct Primary Care?" Dotdash Media.

Ofri, Danielle. "The Patients vs. Paperwork Problem for Doctors." *New York Times*, November 14, 2017.

O'Rourke, Meghan. *The Invisible Kingdom: Reimagining Chronic Illness*. New York: Riverhead Books, 2022.

Pallesen, Jonatan. "Against Scientism." Medium, 2019.

Paris, John J. "Catholic Approaches to End-of-Life Care." *America*, September 22 2015.

Peter G. Peterson Foundation. "How Much Government Spending Goes to Children?" www.pgpf.org/blog/2022/01/how-much-government-spending-goes-to-children.

Press, Matthew J. "Instant Replay—A Quarterback's View of Care Coordination." *New England Journal of Medicine* 371, no. 6 (2014): 489–91.

Reinhardt, Uwe E. *Priced Out: The Economic and Ethical Costs of American Health Care*. Princeton, New Jersey: Princeton University Press, 2019.

Richmond, Caroline. "Dame Cicely Saunders." *British Medical Journal* 331, no. 7510 (2005): 238.

Riley, Gerald F., and James D. Lubitz. "Long-Term Trends in Medicare Payments in the Last Year of Life." *Health Services Research* 45, no. 2 (2010): 565–76.

Robertson, Harry. "Almost a Fifth of All US Dollars Were Created This Year." City A.M. www.cityam.com/almost-a-fifth-of-all-us-dollars-were-created -this-year/.

Robinson, M. K., M. J. DeHaven, and K. A. Koch. "Effects of the Patient Self-Determination Act on Patient Knowledge and Behavior." *Journal of Family Practice* 37, no. 4 (October 1993): 363–68.

Rohr, Richard. "Coming to Terms with Life and Love." Center for Action and Contemplation.

Sallnow, Libby, Richard Smith, Sam H. Ahmedzai, Afsan Bhadelia, Charlotte Chamberlin, Yali Cong, and Brett Doble. "Report of the *Lancet* Commission on the Value of Death: Bringing Death Back Into Life." *Lancet* 399, no. 10327 (February 26, 2022): 837–84.

Sheiner, Louise. "The Long-Term Impact of Aging on the Federal Budget." Washington, DC: Brookings Institution, 2018.

Shrank, William H., Teresa L. Rogstad, and Natasha Parekh. "Waste in the US Health Care System: Estimated Costs and Potential for Savings." *JAMA* 322, no. 15 (2019): 1501–9.

Singleton, Amanda. "What to Know at the Beginning of Your Care Giving Journey." AARP.

Solomon, Sheldon, Jeff Greenberg, and Tom Pyszczynski. *The Worm at the Core: On the Role of Death in Life.* New York: Random House, 2015.

Solzhenitsyn, Alexander. "Harvard Address." 1978.

Sowell, Thomas. *Dismantling America: And Other Controversial Essays.* New York: Basic Books, 2010.

Span, Paula. "For Older Patients, an 'Afterworld' of Hospital Care." *New York Times,* 2019.

Stefan, Susan. *Rational Suicide, Irrational Laws: Examining Current Approaches to Suicide in Policy and Law.* New York: Oxford University Press, 2016.

Sulmasy, Daniel P. "Holding Life and Death in Dynamic Tension." *Health Progress* (November–December 2017).

Taubman, Sarah L., Heidi L. Allen, Bill J. Wright, Katherine Baicker, and Amy N. Finkelstein. "Medicaid Increases Emergency-Department Use: Evidence from Oregon's Health Insurance Experiment." *Science* 343, no. 6168 (2014): 263–68.

Teno, Joan M. "Promoting Multifaceted Interventions for Care of the Seriously Ill and Dying." *JAMA Health Forum* 3, no. 4 (2022).

Thoreau, Henry D. *The Writings of Henry Thoreau, volume 1.* New York: Houghton & Mifflin, 1893.

Tisdale, Sallie. *Advice for Future Corpses (and Those Who Love Them): A Practical Perspective on Death and Dying.* New York: Touchstone Books, 2018.

U.S. Government Accountability Office. "Prescription Drugs: Medicare Spending on Drugs with Direct-to-Consumer Advertising."

Ventola, C. Lee. "Direct-to-Consumer Pharmaceutical Advertising: Therapeutic or Toxic?" *P&T* 36, no. 10 (2011): 669–84.

Volandes, Angelo E. *The Conversation: A Revolutionary Plan for End-of-Life Care.* New York: Bloomsbury Publishing, 2015.

Watkins, David. "Advance Care Planning and Its Impact on Surviving Family Members (and Hospitals)." Mather Institute.

Weiner, Eric. *The Socrates Express: In Search of Life Lessons from Dead Philosophers.* New York: Avid Reader Press, 2020.

Weissman, David. "Policy Proposal: Do Not Resuscitate Orders, a Call for Reform." *Virtual Mentor* 5, no. 1 (January 1, 2003).

Wharton School of the University of Pennsylvania. "Cause and Effect: Do Prescription Drug Ads Really Work?" Knowledge at Wharton. https://knowledge.wharton.upenn.edu/article/prescription-drug-ads/.

Wilkinson, Anne, Neil S. Wenger, and Lisa R. Shugarman. "Advance Directives and Advance Care Planning: Report to Congress." U.S. Department of Health and Human Services, 2008.

Yadav, Kuldeep N., Nicole B. Gabler, Elizabeth Cooney, Saida Kent, Jennifer Kim, Nicole Herbst, Adjoa Mante, Scott D. Halpern, and Katherine R. Courtright. "Approximately One in Three US Adults Completes Any Type of Advance Directive for End-of-Life Care." *Health Affairs* 36, no. 7 (July 1, 2017): 1244–51.

Zitter, Jessica Nutik. *Extreme Measures: Finding a Better Path to the End of Life.* New York: Avery, 2017.

Zuckerman, Jake, and Terry DeMio. "Judge Rules Hospital Must Use Ivermectin: COVID–19 Patient Sought Drug CDC Warns Against." *Cincinnati Enquirer*, August 31, 2021.

INDEX

Aaron, Henry, 127

accessibility, to patients: of AHDs, 119–20; Medicaid impacting, 187; Medicare and, 158–59; of palliative care, 104, 107, 158, 161–62, 182; of PCPs, 136–39, 145–46, 152–53; of telehealth, 144; of videos, 183–84

Accountable Care Organizations (ACOs), 134–35

Accreditation Council for Graduate Medical Education, 38

ACOs. *See* Accountable Care Organizations

advanced care planning (ACP), 114, 216n12; billing codes for, 21–22; for EOL care, 179–80; with PCPs, 118

advance healthcare directives (AHDs), 32, 99, 122, 212; accessibility of, 119–20; Americans lacking, 28, 114; creation of, 118–19; education on, 181; the elderly adopting, 124; Flanagan, M., without, 44; healthcare without, 33; natural death included in, 105–6; nurse violating, 13–14; sentinel events and, 15, 211; Singleton on, 113; surgery avoided by, 56

advertising, for prescription drugs, 169–71

Advice for Future Corpses (Tisdale), 68

AED. *See* automated external defibrillator

Aetna (insurance company), 160

African Americans, hospice care avoided by, 75

After Virtue (MacIntyre), 35

aging: of Americans, 52–53, 94; Cicero on, 95; decline with, 212; detachment required by, 42; EOL and, 194; invisibility and, 93; trade-offs with, 6. *See also* old age

AHDs. *See* advance healthcare directives

Ahmari, Sohrab, 3, 198

Alder Hey Children's Hospital, 77–79

"Alfie's Army" (protest group), 79

Alpert, Abby E., 171

alternative medicine, 139

AMA. *See* American Medical Association

American Board of Internal Medicine, 190

American Medical Association (AMA), 170

Americans, 101, 166; African, 75; aging of, 52–53, 94; AHDs lacked

homecare, hospice care without,
162–63
hospice care, 110, 164; African
Americans avoiding, 75; billing
codes burdening, 160; culture
deprioritizing, 42; curative care
with, 159–60; EOL signaled by,
158; healthcare disconnected from,
157; without homecare, 162–63;
lung transplant compared with,
165; medical necessity and, 161;
palliative care differentiated from,
103–5; patients underutilizing,
166; physicians avoiding, 105;
treatments ended by, 104
hospital, 78; Alder Hey Children's,
77, 79; Bambino Gesù, 78; ICU
at, 65–66; long-term-care, 28–29;
patients emptied from, 77; St.
Joseph, 43–44, 98; St. Mary's, 31,
88, 89. *See also* emergency room
(ER)
Howard, Gregory, 82
How to Grow Old (Cicero), 95

ICD. *See* International Statistical
Classification of Diseases and
Related Health Problems
illness. *See* chronic illness
"immortality projects," Becker on,
84–85
informed consent, 71–73
Institute of Medicine (IOM), 51–52
institutions: dying in, 203; the elderly
isolated in, 93–94; in old age, 25.
See also nursing home
insurance, health, 44, 105, 128, 160;
without billing codes, 148–49;
curative care discouraged by,
54; death trap influenced by, 22;
Gundersen Health System owning,

124; legislation needed for, 152–53;
medical necessity required by,
131, 140; palliative care limited
by, 104, 158–59; patients stymied
by, 129–30; policy excluding,
159; private, 150, 169. *See also*
Medicaid; Medicare; payment
model, insurance; reimbursement,
insurance
intensive care unit (ICU), at hospital,
65–66
International Statistical Classification
of Diseases and Related Health
Problems (ICD), 128
IOM. *See* Institute of Medicine
ivermectin, COVID-19
pandemic and, 81–82

James, Kate, 78
Jefferson, Thomas, 47, 96
The Jefferson Bible (Manseau), 35
Jung, Carl, 93

Kaiser Permanente, 134
Keefe, Patrick Radden, 171
Kevin (patient), 108–11
Kliff, Sarah, 129
Kouwenhoven, William B., 17
Krystofiak, Thom, 36
Kübler-Ross, Elisabeth, 83–84, 91,
157
Kutner, Luis, 114–15

Lakdawalla, Darius N., 171
Lamas, Daniela, 28–29, 61
Lancet Commission, 26, 101, 181,
201–2
Lao Tzu (philosopher), 11, 216n1
laws: death-with-dignity, 106–7;
DNR invalidated by, 19–20;

by, 26, 30; overuse of, 170, 190;
science dominating, 37–39; trade-
offs in, 5, 29. *See also* procedures;
treatments
MedPAC, Medicare and, 188–90
Meier, Diane, 161
Mercy Health (healthcare ministry),
98, 134–35
Merit-Based Payment System (MIPS),
136
"Mettle Health" (YouTube channel),
197
MHB. *See* Medicare Hospice Benefit
Miller, B. J., 197
minorities, healthcare distrusted by, 75
Missouri (state), life support decided
on by, 116
de Montaigne, Michel, 196
Mr. K (patient), 177–78
MWI. *See* Medicare Wage Index
MYCHART (electronic portal), 119

The Name of God is Mercy (Francis),
107
National Institute for Health, Britain
(NIH), 188
National Institute for Health and
Care Excellence (NICE), Britain,
188–89
National Institutes of Health, U.S.
(NIH), 103
Natural Causes (Ehrenreich), 27
natural death, 21; AHD including,
105–6; with comfort care, 9;
compassion protocol through, 86;
declaration of desire for, 118; of
patient, 68–69
necessity, medical. *See* medical
necessity
Neumann, Ann, 11, 25–26, 67
New York Appeals Court, 71

NICE. *See* National Institute for
Health and Care Excellence
NIH. *See* National Institute for
Health, Britain; National Institutes
of Health, U.S.
"No Country for Old Age" (Davis), 94
NPs. *See* nurse practitioners
nurse, AHDs violated by, 13–14
nurse practitioners (NPs), 152
nursing home, 25; David in, 12–14;
family considering, 163; Libby in,
15

Ofri, Danielle, 130
old age: attitude and, 96; as chronic
illness, 203–6; without cure,
9, 185, 192; decline in, 6, 94;
institutions in, 25; wisdom in, 95.
See also the elderly
oncologists, patients grieved by, 64
On Death and Dying (Kübler-Ross),
83
organ transplants, limits on, 185–86
O'Rourke, Kevin, 29
O'Rourke, Meagan, 207
Oster, Michael, Jr., 82
Overtreated (Brownlee), 133
The Oxford Book of Aging (Cole and
Winkler), 94

Palin, Sarah, 216n11
Pallesen, Jonatan, 40
palliative care, 181; accessibility of,
104, 107, 158, 161–62, 182;
assisted suicide reduced by, 107;
healthcare disconnected from, 157;
hospice care differentiated from,
103–5; insurance limiting, 104,
158; physicians considering, 106,
182; reimbursement marginalizing,
161; telehealth improving, 144

care recognized by, 62; insurance excluded by, 159; Patient Protection and Affordable Care Act as, 21, 132, 168; Patient Self-Determination Act in, 80–81, 117; public, 192; recommendations for, 210–11. *See also* reforms, healthcare

POLST. *See* physician orders for life-sustaining treatment

prescription drugs, advertising for, 169–71

Press, Matthew J., 177–78

Price, Tim, 54

primary care physicians (PCPs): accessibility of, 136–39, 145–46, 152–53; ACP with, 118; billing codes complicating, 147–48; care coordination by, 175–78, 180, 210; comfort care not offered by, 196; concierge medicine compared with, 146; education led by, 158; EOL care led by, 180–81, 210; ER contrasted with, 137–38; FFS limiting, 153; payment model for, 147–49; reimbursement of, 136, 137, 148, 149–51; salary of, 151–52

private health insurers, 150, 169

procedures, 128; doctor recommending, 7; education before, 72–73; the elderly injured by, 6–7; EOL care contrasted with, 193; misery increased by, 102. *See also* surgery

Pyszczynski, Tom, 85

Quinlan, Karen Ann, 80

racial disparity, patient autonomy and, 75–76

record, electronic medical, 119–20, 211

recorder, loop (medical device), 144

reforms, healthcare, 134, 173, 207; comfort care funded by, 174; EOL care requiring, 23, 51; MIPS and, 135–36; to payment model, 153–55; Weissman proposing, 62

reimbursement, insurance, 121, 135; capitation and, 134; during COVID-19 pandemic, 129; curative care favored by, 50–51; doctors frustrated by, 131; geography varying, 171–73; palliative care marginalized by, 161; patients influenced by, 168–69; of PCPs, 136, 137, 148, 149–51; of physicians, 21–22, 134; reasonable cost, 148. *See also* billing codes; fee for service; payment model

Reinhardt, Uwe, 55, 168, 194–95

relative value unit (RVU), of CPT, 128

religion, fear subdued by, 85

Renée Rose (nun), 31

Respecting Choices (program), 124–25

retirees, transition for, 98

reverse bucket list, 97–99

right to die, 116–17

Riley, Gerald, 49–50

Roosevelt, Franklin D., 155

RVU. *See* relative value unit

salary, of PCPs, 151–52

Sanders, Bernie, 132

Sanders, Cecily, 104

Schiavo, Terri, 80

medicine, 5, 29; Solzhenitsyn articulating, 198–99; Sowell on, 191

tradition, Ahmari emphasizing, 198

treatments, 121–22; comfort care contrasted with, 8; in curative care, 102; EOL limiting, 74–75; high-tech, 22, 65; hospice care ending, 104; therapeutic, 42–43. *See also* life support; procedures

Tuskegee study, 75

The Unbroken Thread (Ahmari), 3, 198

United Kingdom (UK), 78, 188–89

United Network for Organ Sharing (UNOS), 185–86

United States (U.S.): BLS of, 172; Congress of, 48, 51, 117, 132–36; debt in, 47; healthcare in Britain contrasted with, 188–89; NIH in, 103; Supreme Court of, 80, 116. *See also* Americans

UNOS. *See* United Network for Organ Sharing

urgent care centers, 138–39

ventilator, 43–45, 77–78

videos, educational, 26–27; accessibility of, 183–84; Medicare Part B rebating, 184, 211; surgery explained by, 72

Volandes, Angelo E., 183

"Voluntary ACP" (service), 216n12

Wagshul, Fred, 82

Weissman, David, 62, 182

Welch, Jack, 143

WellSpan Health, 179

will, living. *See* living will

Winkler, Mary G., 94

Wisconsin, 90

The Worm at the Core (Solomon, Greenberg, and Pyszczynski), 85

Young, Robert, 37

Zitter, Jessica Nutik, 23, 158

ABOUT THE AUTHOR

Michael Doring Connelly served as CEO of Mercy Health, one of the nation's largest health systems, from 1994 to 2017. Currently he is CEO emeritus of Mercy Health (now Bon Secours Mercy Health System).

From 1976 to 1989 he served as an executive with the Daughters of Charity National Health System (currently the Ascension Health System). He was a divisional CEO in California and a hospital CEO in Chicago. He has experience with healthcare systems in Germany, the United Kingdom, Denmark, Sweden, and Spain. He has also visited healthcare facilities and orphanages around the world, including Port-au- Prince, Haiti; the Mathare Slums of Nairobi, Kenya; Kingston, Jamaica; Georgetown, Guyana; and Panguma, Sierra Leone.

He has extensive governance experience and has chaired Catholic Charities USA; the Urban League of Greater Southwestern Ohio; the National Catholic Health Association; the Catholic Medical Mission Board; and the healthcare-improvement company Premier. He chaired the United Way for Greater Cincinnati in 2013.

He has published seventeen articles in various healthcare journals and currently lives on Johns Island, South Carolina.